PU
HE
EXPLORED
50 STORIES TO CHANGE THE WORLD

Our titles are also available in a range of electronic formats. To order, or for details of our bulk discounts, please go to our website www.criticalpublishing.com or contact our distributor, NBN International, 10 Thornbury Road, Plymouth PL6 7PP, telephone 01752 202301 or email orders@nbninternational.com.

PUBLIC HEALTH EXPLORED

50 STORIES TO CHANGE THE WORLD

JOHN ASHTON AND LOWELL S LEVIN

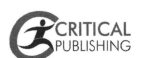

First published in 2021 by Critical Publishing Ltd

British Library Cataloguing in Publication Data
A CIP record for this book is available from the British Library

ISBN: 978-1-913453-93-0
This book is also available in the following e-book formats:

EPUB ISBN: 978-1-913453-95-4
Adobe e-book ISBN: 978-1-913453-96-1

Cover and text design by Fiachra McCarthy
Project management by Newgen Publishing UK
Printed and bound in Great Britain by 4edge, Essex

Critical Publishing
3 Connaught Road
St Albans
AL3 5RX

www.criticalpublishing.com

Paper from responsible sources

DEDICATION

This book is dedicated to Lowell, in absentia, to our wives and families, and to those who work to protect and defend public health wherever they may be.

The health of the people is the highest law.

Cicero

ACKNOWLEDGEMENTS

The short introductory aphorisms at the start of each chapter in this book were all originally published in the *Journal of Epidemiology and Community Health* (JECH) between 2002 and 2007 (www.jech.bmj.com). The authors and publisher would like to express their grateful thanks for permission to use these.

ENDORSEMENT

A fascinating and intriguing book, which has the potential to inspire and instigate debate and argument about the most pressing challenges we face as earthlings. Written with humour, seriousness and experience, it is an essential addition to public health learning and practice.

Richard Lee
Senior Lecturer in Public Health, Northumbria University

CONTENTS

Section 3: Getting started

Section 4: Making a difference

Section 5: Reflections

ABOUT THE AUTHORS

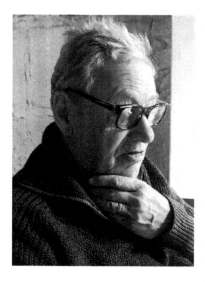

JOHN ASHTON is one of Britain's foremost public health consultants, whose footprint is to be found on many of the most innovative public health initiatives of the past 40 years. Born in Liverpool, John was educated at the University of Newcastle upon Tyne Medical School and the London School of Hygiene and Tropical Medicine, before returning to the northwest where he was a pioneer of the New Public Health. In the 1980s he led work on health promotion, reducing teenage pregnancy, establishing the first large-scale syringe exchange programme in the face of epidemics of heroin injection and the arrival of the human immunodeficiency virus (HIV), and was one of the originators of the World Health Organization (WHO) Healthy Cities Project, now a global programme. John has always bridged the worlds of academia and practice. He is acknowledged as a first-class communicator and inspirational teacher. He has been adviser to the Crown Prince of Bahrain's Covid-19 taskforce and wrote a book on the pandemic. He was awarded the CBE in 2000 for contributions to the NHS.

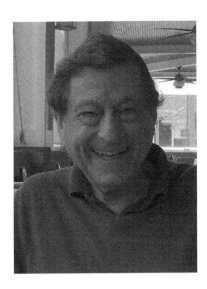

LOWELL S LEVIN (1927–2019), Yale School of Public Health (YSPH) Professor Emeritus, with decades of service to the WHO European Region, as well as the Pan American Health Organization (PAHO), was an inspirational leader in public health, as a teacher, mentor and colleague. Lowell zeroed in on previously unexplored areas such as citizen participation in health and non-professional resources in health care, primarily self-care. Questioning established thought, he brought attention to the pervasiveness of medical errors and pressed for reforms. He was a prominent voice worldwide who fostered cross-disciplinary and intersectoral collaboration to advance awareness of the social and economic determinants of health through examination of a wide range of public policies and their impacts on the public's health. He established the global health programme at the Yale School of Public Health, and initiated numerous health-promoting and educational programmes at local and international levels. Lowell had a lasting impact on students, community leaders, health care practitioners and professionals around the world. In addition to books, Lowell wrote hundreds of journal articles, edited numerous journals, published in news media, offered lectures and seminars for global students and appeared in TV interviews. His wisdom and humour are captured in this book.

LOWELL S LEVIN: A TRIBUTE BY JOANNA STUART

Professor Emeritus Lowell S Levin – Lowell – was a visionary leader in public health. Some concepts in public health accepted today as commonplace became mainstream after Lowell was among the first to express them, at times to great resistance. He showed courage in challenging established health beliefs and practices, always with clear thinking and substantial data. He threw light on the extent of hospital-based medical mistakes and infections, with later studies reaching his same conclusions on the prevalence of these problems. He was also ahead of his time in his early work that linked health to social relations and behaviour. Lowell pioneered the citizen participation movement and brought attention to the role of non-professional resources in strengthening personal capacity for health and well-being, primarily through self-care.

For half a century, Lowell focused on global health, working with the Milbank Memorial Fund, the Pan American Health Organization (PAHO), the WHO European Region, non-governmental organisations, foundations and governmental departments. His work took him to the Caribbean, South America, East Africa and Europe. Lowell was an inspiring communicator in speeches, lectures, conferences, seminars, classes, TV and radio interviews and published works. He also impacted public health thinking through editorships of numerous professional journals and advisory roles in many public and private organisations.

Lowell participated in the development of the Ottawa Charter for Health Promotion (WHO et al, 1986), a historic document that matched Lowell's priorities, such as his commitment to empower local communities, promote healthy public policies and respond to inequities in health, which are inseparable from social, economic and environmental conditions.

Lowell promoted a view of health within the context of social and economic determinants and encouraged policymakers in all sectors to take account of health impacts. Towards this goal, in the first decade of the twenty-first century Lowell collaborated with Erio Ziglio, then director of the WHO European Office for Investment for Health and Development, located in Venice. Together, they offered training programmes to professionals around the world who represented various governmental sectors. These seminars explored how to build healthy public policies within the framework of investment for health.

Attention to health issues as defined by local populations was a critical component of Lowell's thinking, and he was a community activist himself. He believed that listening to people's health concerns and views of how to solve them was crucial. Throughout his career, he continued to think globally and act locally, with an understanding of cultural and social norms. In New Haven, Connecticut, home to Yale, he galvanised a We Mean Clean movement in which he met with residents on Saturday mornings to pick up litter in their neighbourhoods, following the maxim that garbage begets garbage and clean environments remain cleaner. In another local initiative, he organised the clean-up of a rubbish-filled New Haven lagoon. The fresh water was then stocked with fish and became the centre of a new official city public park.

Across the globe, Lowell encouraged approaching problem-solving in new ways, including looking at who defines the problem along with finding solutions revealed within the parameters of the problem itself. He was an entertaining speaker who could deliver his message in a powerful way to impact a listener's understanding. With real life stories, humour, warmth, and always going the extra mile to offer support to those who needed it, Lowell's influence on others was profound. At the same time, he remained humble, rewarded by seeing students on their path

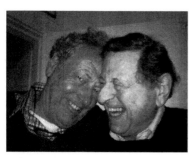

John and Lowell

towards productive careers and by the deep friendships he developed with many of his colleagues, including John Ashton, who was inspired by their work together to write this book. Lowell's great pleasures included lively conversations, great meals and lots of laughter with friends and colleagues, whether hosting international visitors in New Haven or on his own trips abroad. Lowell cared for his professional friends as his family, and feelings were reciprocal.

Lowell S Levin was my husband for 18 years and friend for 30-plus prior years until his death at 91 in 2019. When John Ashton asked me to give my blessing to this book, I felt we were back as a team. John and Lowell's work was fulfilling to both of them, and I carry on Lowell's long friendship with John and his wife, Maggi Morris.

Lowell was a treasure. He saw each person who knew him as special, was genuinely interested in everyone, generous, and ready to help in any way he could. Besides opening his home to students for informal gatherings, he gave personal attention to each student's postgraduate career aims. In 1990 at Yale, he established the Division of International Health and founded its successor, the Global Health Division, in 1994. He encouraged cross-disciplinary studies for public health students, and served as director of the WHO/Yale Collaborating Centre for Health Promotion Policy and Research. Students from the first class to graduate from the Division of International Health reunited after 20 years in a visit at Lowell's home, laden with gifts of appreciation and reminiscences of their beloved professor's contributions to their accomplished careers.

In more than 35 years at Yale, Lowell inspired and guided thousands of students to grow professionally. Years after his retirement, he could barely walk down a street in New Haven without a former student running up to greet him and tell him that they remembered a sentence he once said in class, which they still rely on as a guide in their daily work. To honour Lowell, the Yale University School of Public Health established an annual monetary Lowell S Levin Award in 2009, given to a new graduate dedicated to promoting global health.

For more than a decade during retirement Lowell dedicated himself to an intensive personal challenge in which he voraciously read world literature from centuries past to the present. He enjoyed the aesthetic experience, but also found immersed in these novels many of the public health lessons he had provided over the decades. From conditions of poverty to the spread of diseases, from healing practices and hygienic customs to social and economic inequities, much of world literature painted a picture of public health challenges relevant to our present condition.

Lowell will always be remembered for his intellect, impact, warmth, generosity, respect and care for others, enhanced by his engaging sense of humour.

Joanna G Stuart, PhD, MPH

INTRODUCTION

The use of aphorisms, allegories and stories to influence and educate is as old as the holy books of the great religions and probably older (eg, the pre-literate tradition of Aboriginal storytelling). We learn by observing and doing and by sharing experiences; using stories and parables to communicate abstract ideas in tangible ways.

The idea for this book grew out of the publication of a series of curated aphorisms by the authors in the *Journal of Epidemiology and Community Health* (JECH) between 2002 and 2007. This section of the journal was well-received at the time with feedback, especially from teachers of public health, that the aphorisms were a valuable resource in the classroom.

Although Lowell and I discussed the possibility of gathering together a collection of the most salient examples into a small book, the demands of everyday life meant that the project never reached the top of the pile before Lowell's death at the age of 91 in 2019. The irony of this lies in the heart of one of Lowell's aphorisms: that the way to tackle multiple tasks is to construct a list in a hierarchy, running from the easiest to the most difficult, beginning at the top and working down. In this way a momentum is established in which the feedback loop of success enables progression through to the most difficult challenge.

This project should have always been at the top of the list, as we had already done most of the hard work in capturing the stories brought together here. It took the joyous celebration of Lowell's contribution to public health, and the thousands of former students for whom he had been such an important figure in their personal and professional development in New Haven, to galvanise me into action.

I first met Lowell in Copenhagen in 1986. I had been invited by the World Health Organization to be part of a group to plan the Healthy Cities Project under the leadership of rising star Ilona Kickbusch. That project would turn out to be a global phenomenon which is still going strong 35 years later, involving thousands of cities in national networks. Lowell, a major figure in international public health, an inspirational professor at the Yale School of Public Health and a generous mentor from an older generation, was a regular visitor to Copenhagen where his wise guidance impacted many of us.

Over the ensuing years Lowell, his first wife Corinne, and later his second wife Joanna, became close friends with frequent visits between New Haven, Liverpool and later Dent. Lowell's early morning appearances at Manchester Airport, always first off the plane with his small, battered suitcase, became part of his legend. After a short pri-esta he was up and raring to go with a combination of zest, passion, humour and anecdote that kept any audience gagging for more. His 'An Evening with Lowell S Levin' could have kept many audiences going all night and for all of us this became part of an ongoing seminar of a shared passion for public health lasting more than 30 years.

Tragically, Corinne's early death from a brain tumour ended a remarkable partnership in which Corinne's lifetime of developmental work with childminders from communities in New England so complemented Lowell's commitment to the disadvantaged. Fortunately, when Lowell renewed his acquaintance with Joanna, herself recently widowed, a new life was created for both and Joanna's background in anthropology and public health brought new riches to bear.

Many of the best teachers are great storytellers, always filling a room and thinking on their feet. This was Lowell in a nutshell. Between 1998 and 2008 I had the privilege of co-editing the *Journal of Epidemiology and Community Health* with my dear friend and colleague Professor Carlos Alvarez-Dardet, from Seville and Alicante, with the support of Maggi Morris, Sonia McKeown and Miguel Porta. During this period Lowell and I began to curate regular aphorisms for publication in JECH to illustrate public health in action, and it is these that form the basis of this new volume.

I hope that you find nourishment in this collection, which I offer in memory of a very dear friend and colleague in the year of the Covid-19 pandemic. Many of these aphorisms have special salience this year; if Lowell was still with us there would have been more.

John Ashton, 2021
Dent and Liverpool

SECTION 1
CONCEPTS

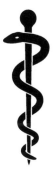

APHORISM 1: DEFINING THE PROBLEM

The person who defines the problem controls the range of solutions.

JECH, July 2005, 59: 597

Public health problems are rarely simple and depend on the perspective of the person defining them. They are usually multifactorial and require different approaches depending on the desired outcome.

FOR DISCUSSION

+ Can they be prevented completely? Do they need to be managed in the optimal way to reduce harm, or do we have to learn to live with them?
+ In any event, what harms are we talking about – the purely medical such as disability and death, or wider social and economic harms; and who do the harms most affect?
+ Who has the loudest voice in deciding what is important and what is the evidence being deployed?

CASE STUDY

The Covid-19 pandemic demonstrates many of these dilemmas. At the beginning of the pandemic there was a reluctance by China to share what was happening with the world community and diplomatic considerations led the World Health Organization (WHO) to hold off calling it a pandemic. In the United Kingdom, the government of the day was distracted by the impending exit from the European Union (Brexit) and the prime minister by complex matters in his personal life.

In this case, the framing of the outbreak in China as not being a concern in Western countries led to the loss of precious time; once the urgency was better understood, its framing as primarily a medical and hospital issue led to insufficient attention being given to the wider public health agenda of public mobilisation, building capacity for self and community care, including family medicine to reduce the need for hospitalisation, and the threat to those of vulnerable status in institutional settings, such as care homes and prisons.

Delay in taking the threat to public health seriously and a top-down approach which was politically framed led to a failure to get to grips with the need to massively increase the capacity for testing for the virus and to hand control of testing to local public health teams. Failure to be open and transparent with the public and of senior figures to set an example led to a breakdown of trust, compromising adherence to the need for self-discipline in adopting mask-wearing and social distancing when the epidemic underwent a resurgence.

The consequence of all these failings was thousands of avoidable deaths and catastrophic damage to the nation's economy in the United Kingdom (Ashton, 2020).

_____

APHORISM 2: ON FORGETTING YOUR PRINCIPLES

Sometimes it is necessary to forget your principles and do the right thing.

JECH, April 2004, 58: 264

FOR DISCUSSION

+ What are the values that underpin the practice of public health and how have these varied over time in different communities and places?
+ What are the professional obligations of public health professionals when their own beliefs conflict with the legal framework of the country in which they are working?
+ How should such conflicts be handled?

CASE STUDY

In contemporary societies with complex mixtures of peoples, races and faiths, finding common ground in contentious matters involving personal behaviour that impacts on others or on the environment that sustains us can be difficult. Early laws for communal life are to be found in the great religions. Later, philosophers endeavoured to make sense of the need for ethical frameworks in an increasingly secular world, stressing such concepts as respect for autonomy, proportionality and adherence to rules that are for the common good (Seedhouse, 2001).

In nineteenth-century public health, one of the most influential voices was that of the utilitarian moral philosopher Jeremy Bentham, who espoused the cause of '*the greatest good of the greatest number*', and John Stuart Mill, who wrote that '*Freedom only deserves that name as long as it doesn't deprive others of theirs*'; perhaps most succinctly expressed colloquially in the American claim that '*Your freedom ends where my nose begins*' (Mill, 1859).

Often the most contentious issues in public health lie in the complex area between personal behaviour and traditional or longstanding cultural attitudes and beliefs such as those relating to personal and sexual relationships, marital and family obligations, and adherence to the laws of the land, such as those relating to the use of illicit drugs. Since the Second World War, attitudes in many of these areas have been in flux with a progressive trend towards the recognition of more individual choices and a loosening of the bounds of tradition to be found in religion.

During the 1970s and 1980s, following the introduction of the contraceptive pill, there was a revolution in the acceptance of different sexual norms in many countries, with same-sex relationships becoming accepted by most people, sex outside marriage becoming normalised and safe abortion becoming available in response to women's desire to control their own childbearing options. Finding a path between those with traditional values and those demanding greater autonomy was not always easy and for public health pragmatic considerations, focusing on individual and group health and well-being, came to the fore.

In the 1980s the triple threat of high levels of youth unemployment, an epidemic of injection heroin abuse, together with a highly infectious new virus – HIV, causing the disease of AIDS by sexual and body fluid transmission including via injection – brought some of these issues together. This resulted in pilots of large-scale syringe exchange programmes to ensure that heroin and other drug injectors were not put at risk by sharing syringes. The success of this approach in keeping the human immunodeficiency virus (HIV) from spreading in this population led to it being adopted internationally and spawning a new concept in the practice of public health, known as 'harm reduction' in which people who may have been opposed to a behaviour in principle found it necessary to *forget their principles and do the right thing* (Ashton and Seymour, 1989; Ashton, 2019).

APHORISM 3: THE WORLD IS A FAST FLOWING RIVER

The world is a fast flowing river.

JECH, January 2003, 57: 2

One of the powerful aphorisms in giving shape to the New Public Health movement in the 1980s was that the world was a fast flowing river, with health care workers standing on the banks with white water swirling below. Every so often a drowning person would be swept down and our workers/life-savers would jump in, pull them out and resuscitate them. They were so busy jumping in, pulling out and resuscitating that they had no time to walk upstream and see who was pushing everybody in (Ashton and Seymour, 1989).

FOR DISCUSSION

✚ Can you give three examples of public health issues where the emphasis is predominantly on downstream interventions when there are upstream measures that would save people from being at risk of drowning?
✚ What kind of evidence do you need to make the case for a change of emphasis to upstream action?
✚ Why do you think it is so difficult to reorientate health services towards a greater emphasis on public health and prevention?
✚ What examples are there where these efforts have been successful and why has success been possible?

CASE STUDY

This metaphor resonates with the everyday claims of clinicians that they are too busy to focus on prevention. At the same time it raises questions about the policies that might keep people away from the river in the first place – environmental measures of fences, warning notices and other measures to keep people from falling or jumping in; lifestyle measures such as swimming lessons; and the appropriate balance between early assistance from lifeguards or later support from emergency ambulances and casualty departments. Without a balanced approach all the resources could be focused downstream.

A paradox of the dominance of treatment over prevention in health is that measures that may prevent a disease or condition from leading to death can lead to an increased burden of a disease by increasing its prevalence in the community.

In the case of type II diabetes mellitus, for example, with its association with obesity, medical treatment can reduce the morbidity but lead to the accumulation of very large numbers of patients in the community who require a lifetime of care, medication and support and may still require a variety of specialist interventions to deal with the long-term complications. This can be largely avoided by the maintenance of a healthy weight and lifestyle.

APHORISM 4: ELEPHANTS ON A TRAIN IN AFRICA

There is a story of two people travelling on a train in Africa. One of them is throwing powder out of the window. Her puzzled travelling companion asks her what she is doing. She replies that she is throwing powder out of the window to keep the elephants away. 'There are no elephants', replies the inquisitor. 'There you are', retorts the powder-thrower, 'it works!'

JECH, October 2002, 56: 721

FOR DISCUSSION

✚ Can you give three examples of problems that are out of sight and out of mind such that prevention is ignored or neglected?
✚ Why do you think that there is institutional and professional resistance to prioritising issues of this kind?
✚ What strategies and approaches might be adopted to make the invisible visible and ensure that such issues receive the attention they deserve?

CASE STUDY

The problem with prevention is that things, once prevented, become invisible. Somehow, public health must make visible and real those threats to public health that have apparently been consigned to history but may return causing serious threats to health and well-being. The Danish poet and polymath Piet Hein captures this in one of his 'grook' poems: *'problems worthy of attack prove their worth by hitting back'* (Hein, 1969).

This challenge of making the invisible visible is particularly applicable to the infectious diseases that used to cause such a toll of misery, ill health and death but which have been dramatically reduced in many countries as a result of improvements in standards of living and environments. However, they may still be lurking in the wings, waiting to return given appropriate circumstances.

Childhood infections such as measles, mumps, rubella, whooping cough, diphtheria and polio are examples of diseases that used to kill significant numbers of children three or four generations ago but have become uncommon as a result of effective programmes of immunisation and vaccination. Vaccination coverage rates have been adversely affected in many countries as a result of ill-informed and crank-led hostility to these programmes, potentially putting children at risk.

In recent years we have experienced the appearance of a series of novel virus infections, including avian flu, SARS, swine flu, Ebola and now Covid-19, that have jumped from species that were adapted to them to humans who have no resistance. These developments may have occurred as a result of extensive urbanisation and the encroachment of slum areas into virgin areas that are the natural habitats of other species.

It is essential to maintain constant vigilance for the emergence or re-emergence of outbreaks of infectious diseases. Keeping the public abreast of these threats to health and the importance of protecting themselves and their loved ones requires the building of a trusting relationship between health professionals and the community and imaginative approaches to open and transparent communications making use of all media modalities as well as cultural activities such as drama in education, soap opera plots on radio and television and the sharing of real life stories and experiences. By such means it will be possible to keep the elephants away.

APHORISM 5: ELEPHANTS AND THE PREVENTION OF INFANT DEATHS

There is a parable about an international agency working in a rural area of Asia where infant mortality rates are very high, often associated with infantile diarrhoea. The development team decide that what is needed is to improve sanitation in the village and they install a communal latrine block. Some years later they revisit the area and find that the latrines are unused and broken and that the health situation remains much the same. Somebody suggests that they should find out from the villagers what has gone on and what they think about it all.

What they discover is that it is not that the villagers are uncaring about the fate of their children but that sanitation is not at the top of their list of priorities. Their major preoccupation is that every year when the sugar cane is nearly ready the elephants appear and trample it down so the villagers cannot harvest it and obtain economic benefit. As a result of the discussions a new project is undertaken to protect the sugar from the elephants. When this is proved to be successful the credibility of the international group is enhanced and the villagers are ready to talk about other concerns including infant welfare and sanitation.

JECH, November 2002, 56: 802

FOR DISCUSSION

+ Can you give an example where it has been difficult to engage with a community but it has subsequently been possible to find common ground and work together on an issue?
+ What do you see as the main issues in establishing common ground and overcoming obstacles?

CASE STUDY

I discovered this truth for myself in the Liverpool inner city area of Vauxhall in the early 1980s, an old Irish working-class area of the city. The Eldon Street Community Association had organised themselves when the city council had threatened to demolish their houses as part of slum clearance. The Eldonians' motto was '*Professionals should be on tap, not on top*' and they had clear priorities for their community, beginning with decent housing, good schools for the children and a safe neighbourhood. With far and away the worst health statistics in the city, poorly served by medical services, sky-high smoking rates and an appalling diet, these things took second place to their own clear understanding of what needed to be achieved first. Thirty years later with their priorities largely met, this community is heavily engaged in the health promotion and improvement activities that had preoccupied health professionals so many years earlier (McBane, 2008).

APHORISM 6: EATING AN ELEPHANT

It is said that the thing about eating an elephant is that it doesn't much matter where you start, the important thing is to know that it is indeed an elephant, and that you have some sense of its size and shape, and where the hard bits and the fleshy bits are.

JECH, December 2002, 56: 887

FOR DISCUSSION

+ Can you give an example of a public health problem that is complex and which people tend to put in the 'too difficult' box?
+ How might you identify entry points which would make it possible to make a start and 'get a face' on the issue?
+ Can you identify the forces for progress and the obstacles in making a start?

CASE STUDY

As with elephants, so with public health. The determinants of public health range far and wide, from the environment through culture and behaviour, biology, social and political institutions and all the settings where we live, love, work and play. If we are not to be paralysed by the enormity of the challenge, we do need a picture, a map, a sense of the jigsaw. How often have you been told that it is all too big and complex and that you should focus down on one or two initiatives?

In work for public health there is a major tension between having comprehensive strategies and achieving piecemeal progress in the daily round. Of course we must do both; without an understanding of the big picture and a 'strategic underview' how can serendipity favour the prepared mind? How can we be strategically opportunistic when the opportunity presents itself?

In the 1980s, teenage pregnancy loomed large on the public health radar. In Liverpool, with a large Roman Catholic population and half the schools being faith-based, there was a prevalent view in the Health Authority that it would not be possible to ensure that sex and relationships education was provided in each school. However, the Catholic hierarchy had never been asked. When the Archbishop was approached it was discovered that he believed that there *should* be such education to ensure that young people had the biological knowledge while the church would provide the religious and ethical values (Ashton, 2019).

APHORISM 7: THE AGE OF HYGIEIA

It is time that we replaced public health's aggressive disease-orientated Aesculapius symbol of medicine with the more peaceful countenance of Hygieia, who more accurately reflects the commitment to public health

JECH, August 2007, 61: 712

In Greek mythology Aesculapius, the god of medicine, had several daughters, including Hygieia and Panacea. For the worshippers of Hygieia, health was the natural order of things, something that people could expect if they lived their lives wisely. In contrast, the followers of Panacea were more sceptical, believing that people were intrinsically foolish and liable to neglect their health, in which case the role of the physician was to correct imperfections and imbalances resulting from disturbances of the body's natural balance.

FOR DISCUSSION

✚ What examples can you give where Panacea rules the roost and Hygieia would stand a much better chance of ensuring health and well-being?

✚ Why do you think people are so drawn to worship at the feet of Panacea and to ignore the teachings of Hygieia?

✚ What are the levers available to public health to shift the balance more towards Hygieia?

CASE STUDY

Road traffic accidents are a major cause of premature death and disability around the world. In the early days of the motor car, such events were remarkably common as growth in the numbers of vehicles meant that populations needed to adapt to their presence in familiar environments and learned to cope with their unaccustomed speed. Something similar occurred with the early days of the steam engine, when British government's President of the Board of Trade William Huskisson became the first fatality of the new method of transport in 1830. Huskisson misjudged the speed of the famous Rocket steam engine on its trials between Liverpool and Manchester and fell under its wheels; it was travelling at around ten miles per hour.

With motoring increasingly becoming available to the masses, resulting in an annual total of 7,343 road traffic deaths in 1934, minister of transport Leslie Hore-Belisha set about introducing a series of measures to make the roads safer, especially for pedestrians who made up half the victims. Hore-Belisha's Road Traffic Act of 1934 set a speed limit of 30 miles per hour in built-up areas. He subsequently rewrote the Highway Code as the basis of a driving test which he introduced, and established flashing 'Belisha beacons' to demarcate safe crossing areas for pedestrians to negotiate their way safely across busy roads. In these initiatives Hore-Belisha provides us with evidence that parliament is the dispensary of public health.

In subsequent years, improvements in motor car design led to further steady reductions in the death rates especially of car drivers. In the 1960s a major further safety measure was the introduction of seat belts. Initial efforts to persuade the motoring public to adopt their use through educational and advertising campaigns led to little success and eventually further legislation led to their wearing becoming compulsory.

APHORISM 8: WILLIAM MORRIS ON HEALTH

At least I know this, that if a person is overworked in any degree they cannot enjoy the sort of health I am speaking of; nor if they are continually chained to one dull round of mechanical work with no hope at the other end of it; nor if they live in continual sordid anxiety for their livelihood; nor if they are deprived of all enjoyment of the natural beauty of the world; nor if they have no amusement to quicken the flow of their spirits from time to time; all these things, which touch more or less directly on their bodily condition, are born of the claim I make to live in good health (William Morris, 1884).

JECH, November 2003, 57: 887

FOR DISCUSSION

✚ William Morris' definition of health is very broad and inclusive. Do you agree with it or do you find it to be too utopian and all-inclusive?

✚ What other definitions of health are you familiar with?

✚ What are the implications of adopting a broad definition of health, such as that of William Morris, for efforts to improve and protect the health of the population?

CASE STUDY

The Victorian public health movement came about as a result of the crisis of health in the urban slums of the rapidly growing cities of the Industrial Revolution. The initial focus of that movement was on sanitation and the urban environment, with efforts being made to improve slum housing, provide safe water and sewerage, pave the streets and clear them of animal and vegetable matter.

That first phase gave way to an era of hygiene and personal prevention in the 1870s, made possible by the germ theory of disease, household access to soap and water, and later the beginnings of immunisation and vaccination together with family planning. These advances were accompanied by the development of community nursing, health visiting and school health services, as well as important social welfare measures such as the introduction of free school milk and meals. Taken together with general improvements in the standard of living of poorer people and advances in agriculture that reduced the price of food there were significant impacts on death rates from infectious diseases including childhood infections and tuberculosis by the time of the Second World War.

When the war was over the promise held out by early discoveries in pharmaceuticals, such as insulin and penicillin, transformed expectations and led to the belief that public health had largely completed its historic task and that the future would be one of hospitals, clinics and treatments with scientifically derived medicines. Public health in many countries went into a decline until the 1970s when the escalating costs of the diseases of ageing, of long-term conditions and of expensive hospital-based care led to a renewed interest in prevention, in primary health care in the community and in public health.

The 1946 World Health Organization definition of health as *'A complete state of physical, mental and social wellbeing and not merely the absence of disease'* began to attract increasing attention and led to the development of what came to be known as the New Public Health (WHO, 1946; Ashton and Seymour, 1989). The 1946 definition of health was much criticised for being utopian and difficult to operationalise. It was succeeded by a more pragmatic approach in the WHO *Global Strategy for Health for All by the Year 2000*, in which *'The main goal of governments and WHO in coming decades should be the attainment by all citizens of the world by the year 2000 of a level of health that will permit them to lead a socially and economically productive life'* (WHO, 1981).

The WHO *Global Strategy for Health for All by the Year 2000* galvanised a generation of public health and health policy workers to focus on the broader and upstream determinants of health, particularly the attainment of specific targets relating to particular health issues. While progress was made towards many of these targets, others were missed and there was always the danger of hitting the target and missing the point. For philosopher David Seedhouse, health was seen to be *'The foundations of achievement'*, a state of well-being that enabled the realisation of each individual's potential (Seedhouse, 2001).

After the millennium had passed, the WHO went through further iterations of a targeted approach to health improvement and in 2015 the adoption of the United Nations *2030 Agenda for Sustainable Development*, and its Sustainable Development Goals, provided an opportunity for the WHO to embed its public health goals within the more comprehensive imperatives of concerns for global warming and the sustainability of the planet (United Nations, 2015).

APHORISM 9: 'DOING HEALTH': RECLAIMING THE 'H' WORD

Mark Twain famously said that he had been writing prose for 20 years before he knew that that was what he was doing. It is the same with health. Health is created and lost in everyday life by individuals, families and organisations in the settings where people live, love, work and play (Ashton, 1991).

JECH, March 2004, 58: 198

FOR DISCUSSION

✚ Who is responsible for protecting and improving the health of the population?
✚ Why is public health too important to be left only to people with *health*, *medicine* or *clinical* in their job title?
✚ Why do you think that the medical care system finds it so difficult to engage in public health and why do others with significant potential influence over health not realise their potential?

CASE STUDY

The reluctance of people from many different sectors to admit that they are involved in work for health puzzled me for years. One day the penny dropped. The medicalisation of health has led to a linguistic impasse in which health care workers claim to be doing health while predominantly concerning themselves with treating disease, while those actually doing health are reluctant to admit it for fear of being put under the direction of clinical workers.

The Victorian public health movement and the organisational forms that it took in many countries placed the leadership role with physicians and hierarchies presided over by doctors. As the arrangements for public health developed and services grew around them, other professionals such as community and public health nurses, environmental health officers and social workers began to demand their autonomy and separate identities.

In the course of time the challenge of developing a multidisciplinary approach was met with the hiving off of specialist silos and the fragmentation of effort together with a reluctance to own up to being involved in public health for fear of being brought back under medical direction.

For increasingly specialised clinicians, especially those in hospitals, having created their own hierarchies separate from public health, there was no going back to the days when Medical Officers of Health held sway over their local hospital. For the public, the relevance of public health had been eclipsed by the rise of hospital medicine; in addition there was an emerging narrative that equated public health messages as being part of a 'nanny state' that wished to curtail the newfound personal liberties of the post-war years, a narrative that sought to play down the negative forces in play in the form of the commercial determinants of ill health.

We need to reclaim the 'H' word to make it legitimate for non-medical staff and a range of professions allied to medicine to be seen to be in the lead on many health protecting and promoting activities. At the same time we should explore the opportunities for health care workers to contribute to the broad sweep of public health in addition to their roles in disease management.

APHORISM 10: FORESEEING AND FORESTALLING

Man has lost the capacity to foresee and to forestall, he will end by destroying the world.

JECH, May 2003, 57: 314

FOR DISCUSSION

✚ In what ways does the sanitary idea that lay behind the Victorian public health movement differ from the ecological idea that has emerged in recent years?

✚ What are the implications for public health practice that follow from the adoption of an ecological perspective?

✚ What recent initiatives have adopted an ecological approach to global policies for health and the environment?

CASE STUDY

In the 1950s, when he wrote the words above on the ecological crisis facing the planet, Albert Schweitzer was regarded by many as at least eccentric, if not worse, despite the recent experience of global conflict and the use of nuclear weapons. He was writing at about the same time that Watson and Crick were discovering the double helical structure of DNA, and when Rachel Carson was publishing her book *Silent Spring*, which predicted the ecological catastrophe to come (Watson, 1968; Carson, 1962).

Since then little has happened to distract us from the salient truth that how we manage the planet and how we manage relations between ourselves are the two things on which eventually the security of health, well-being and the survival of the human species depend. The evidence for global warming, bringing with it the threat of rising sea levels and the displacement of large populations from low-lying countries, has brought into focus the extent to which international collaboration is essential if we are to bequeath a habitable planet to our grandchildren. There is no Planet B.

As the world again dissolves into global conflicts which are likely to be exacerbated by competition for habitable space and natural resources, including food and water, with the resulting mass migration, we are reminded that public health must be involved in these most central questions.

In 1972 the United Nations Conference on the Human Environment led to the establishment of the World Commission on Environment and Development (WCED) in 1983. The WCED defined sustainable development as '*meeting the needs of the present without compromising the ability of future generations to meet their own needs*'. This definition underpinned the deliberations at the first United Nations Conference on Environment and Development in Rio de Janeiro in 1992 resulting in what became known as 'Agenda 21' and, in the year 2000, the Millennium Development Goals. When those goals expired in 2015 they were replaced by a set of 17 Sustainable Development Goals for the year 2030. These comprehensive goals provide an umbrella for action by all member states of the UN together with local and regional levels of political governance. Three of them in particular, 'Good health and well-being', 'Reduced inequalities', and 'Sustainable cities and communities' have been adopted to be at the heart of the WHO Healthy Cities Project (Ashton, 2019).

The United Nations Sustainable Development Goals

1. No poverty
2. Zero hunger
3. Good health and well-being
4. Quality education
5. Gender equality
6. Clean water and sanitation
7. Affordable and clean energy
8. Decent work and economic growth
9. Industry, innovation, and infrastructure
10. Reduced inequalities
11. Sustainable cities and communities
12. Responsible consumption and production
13. Climate action
14. Life below water
15. Life on land
16. Peace, justice, and strong institutions
17. Partnerships for the goals.

SECTION 2
ISSUES

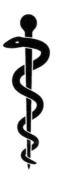

APHORISM 11: A FISH IS THE LAST ONE TO SEE THE WATER

A fish is the last one to see the water.

JECH, June 2007, 61: 498

FOR DISCUSSION

+ What threats can you identify to public health that are so much part of everyday life they are often overlooked?
+ Can you give historical examples of such threats and how they were successfully tackled and eliminated?
+ What are the obstacles to overcoming such ubiquitous threats?

CASE STUDY

In recent times, damaging lifestyles, behaviours and living and working conditions were so prevalent that they were overlooked and regarded as normal. These included tobacco smoking, excessive alcohol consumption, foods high in fat, sugar and salt, sedentary living, road traffic accidents, car exhaust pollution, violence and domestic abuse, excessive working hours, job insecurity and poverty wages.

Commercial interests spend vast amounts of resources diverting us from focusing on the waters that surround us and perpetuating inequalities in health that affect those with less possibility of exerting healthy choices in their lives (Marmot et al, 2010; Kickbusch et al, 2016).

If the fish are the last ones to see the water, one of the key tasks of public health practitioners is to make the invisible visible using all the tools at their disposal. Among these tools are the collection and analysis of data, the rich repertoire of communications and insights that can be derived from the deployment of storytelling, the arts, drama, soap operas and musical art forms. Conventional public health communications such as talks, lectures, and the use of mass and new media are all important in establishing a rapport between expert and lay public and building trust. Intelligence gathering and communications are the bookends of public health.

During the Covid-19 pandemic in the United Kingdom there was a failure to optimise communications. A vendetta against the BBC by Prime Minister Boris Johnson led to a delay in public engagement with a trusted professional voice at the national level, and when it came it failed on the tests of openness and transparency with chaotic political messaging and manipulation of the data for testing and tracing for the virus and in particular the toll of deaths from the virus in various settings and groups of the population. Initially the local Directors of Public Health were prevented from engaging with their populations through the local mainstream and social media, denying them the space to build their relationship with the public and support local people in adopting difficult measures to contain the pandemic.

APHORISM 12: NOT INVENTED HERE

When you come up with all those wonderful ideas for changing the world you will first be told 'It won't work'. When you ask why and say it has worked in Amsterdam, New York, and Gateshead they will tell you 'Yes, but it won't work here'. If you ask if it has been tried here they will say 'No, but it won't work here' and when you ask for an explanation you will be told that to understand why it will require a detailed knowledge of the local culture and history and that this will take some time. At the root of this frustrating encounter will be that 'It wasn't invented here'.

JECH, July 2002, 56: 481

FOR DISCUSSION

+ Why do you think that there is often a reluctance to follow innovation and best practice from elsewhere?
+ Can you give examples of where this has happened to the detriment of public health?
+ What strategies and tactics might you deploy to import and implement effectively public health interventions from elsewhere?

CASE STUDY

The Bible tells us that prophets are not recognised in their own country. It drives politicians mad that good practice and innovation found in one place will not be replicated elsewhere but politicians themselves are not exempt from this weakness.

Various factors may be in play in this situation including ignorance, insecurity, hubris, xenophobia or core personality attributes such as resistance to change. Older personnel may have particular difficulty in accepting that patterns of work that they pioneered in their younger days are now past their sell-by date and be sceptical that not all change is for the best; younger colleagues may be keen to innovate for its own sake to make a mark.

Sometimes a reluctance to follow where the evidence leads can appear to be just perverse. Plagiarism in public health is not a crime as it is in public examinations; rather we should award recognition to those who can take another's innovation and improve on it.

Finding ways into breaking this vicious circle of adherence to often dysfunctional practice requires all the tools of change management. In recent years the main tool for innovation and change has come to be seen as evidence-based practice in which the randomised controlled trial is regarded as the gold standard. However, human populations living in diverse communities are not the same as rat populations in laboratory cages and drawing conclusions based on limited data is often necessary. Even when an accumulation of evidence points in the direction of an intervention endowing benefit there can be resistance to adopting a particular measure.

As home-grown prophets may be ignored, sometimes it is valuable to bring in an expert from outside who has the charisma to persuade local people of the value of a new approach but outsiders may also arouse antibodies. The bottom line is ownership. Whatever approaches are used, communities and communities of interest need to own processes of change and innovation if they are to work and be sustainable.

During the Covid-19 pandemic of 2020, the wearing of masks and face coverings was widely followed in some countries such as China and Japan but initially resisted in others, especially the UK and the United States. In Asia there was a longstanding tradition of face coverings being used by those with respiratory infections which dated from the influenza pandemic of 1918/19. This had been so incorporated into particular cultures to the extent that it is regarded as bad manners to sneeze in public or not wear a mask if you have a respiratory virus.

In some Western countries the reluctance to wear masks may be especially pronounced among men, perhaps due to being seen as not masculine behaviour and there may also be elements of xenophobia. Despite steadily accumulating evidence of the benefits of masks and face coverings during the course of the pandemic some medical advisers to the British government opposed them and in the United States President Trump was actively hostile, probably contributing to the country's large death toll from the virus.

One aspect of the limitations of an evidence-based approach to public health threats is the tendency of professionals to adopt a 'scientistic' attitude to the sharing of knowledge with communities, overwhelming them with graphs and statistics on the assumption that their scientific authority will automatically carry them over the line with little effort to put themselves in the recipient of the knowledge's shoes. Empathy, trust and citizen science are key elements of taking the public on a journey in a public health emergency.

APHORISM 13: LISTEN TO THE COMMUNITY

Listen to the community: it's defining its own problems and may well know what to do about them.

JECH, November 2007, 61: 932

FOR DISCUSSION

+ Can you think of an example when the 'experts' were at odds with a community over the nature of a threat to their well-being and what needed to be done about it?
+ What do you think lies behind the tensions that can exist between these different ways of seeing the world?
+ How can the gap between experts and citizens be bridged?

CASE STUDY

The aphorism from clinical medicine that you should listen to the patient, because they are telling you the diagnosis, is well known. In public health, taking a careful and detailed history of the community issues should contribute to a more valuable diagnosis and effective intervention in the same way. It will also help to avoid paternalistic, top-down and exploitative approaches such as some of the dangers inherent in a naive approach to social marketing or management consultancy.

The charge made against management consultants is that they 'borrow your watch to tell you the time'. Good public health consultants are more like coaches, bringing out inherent strengths.

Following the Grenfell Tower fire in West London in 2017, which claimed the lives of 72 people, there was a complete breakdown of trust between the survivors, bereaved and local residents and the local council and other agencies who were held to be responsible for the fire and for dealing with the aftermath.

A matter that became of particular contention was the failure to test for potentially toxic products of combustion in the environment surrounding the tower in the days and weeks following the fire. The argument put forward by Public Health England (PHE) for not implementing enhanced environmental surveillance, including soil sampling, was that the plume from the fire had ascended vertically and was taken away by the prevailing wind. Enhanced monitoring of the air was not put in place for more than ten days, and in the absence of findings PHE rejected the necessity of soil sampling to the anger of local people who had experienced significant fallout of combustion 'char' from the burnt tower and its fabric.

In a battle between the 'scientistic' assertions of the experts and the citizen science of the local residents, trust was an enduring casualty. In the absence of adequate capacity for soil toxicology in the local authority a Scientific Advisory Group was established under the government Chief Scientist to oversee a programme of testing. This was something it embarked on with reluctance, leading to the resignation from the group of a leading international authority on combustion toxicology and the further entrenchment of suspicion and alienation of the community.

APHORISM 14: BEWARE OF HEALTHISM

Beware of healthism.

JECH, May 2005, 59: 370

FOR DISCUSSION

+ What do you think is meant by the idea of 'healthism'?
+ Do you agree that health as a goal trumps other aspirations that people may have for what they wish to get out of life?
+ What other priorities are in competition for attention in comparison to health goals?

CASE STUDY

For most people health is not life's goal and is taken for granted until it is compromised. Public health is not a religion although sometimes the passion that public health workers have for their vocation can give that impression. It is a journey rather than a destination. Health is a means to an end, a resource for a full life, well lived, rather than something to be obsessively pursued in a way that denies the enjoyment and management of risk and testing limits (Seedhouse, 2001).

There is a danger in public health that those who are drawn to work in this area may assume that everybody shares their enthusiasm such that it overrides the ethical principle of respect for autonomy. At its extreme, such as in Nazi Germany in the 1930s, this can become part of a totalitarian ideology.

On the other hand, extreme libertarians, who are often to be found in the company of dogmatic free marketeers, may argue that the state has no business interfering with individual citizens' life choices freely made.

The tension between prioritising the prevention of deaths from Covid-19 and the impact of locking down everyday life to stop the circulation of the coronavirus was played out on a daily basis during the pandemic of 2020 (Ashton, 2020).

Around the world economies ground to a halt as measures were put in place to stop the movement and mixing of people to reduce the conditions favouring the spread of the virus. At times there seemed to be a false dichotomy between protecting public health and protecting the economy.

If this false dichotomy is allowed to dominate public discourse there may be no winners. On the contrary, providing conditions in which the public is safe and secure can enable the pursuit of individual liberty and a dynamic economy. Those countries that took prompt action during the Covid-19 pandemic not only experienced far fewer Covid deaths but also generally had economies that proved to be more resilient than those in which governments took a hands-off approach.

In addition, the constraints on everyday life brought about by requiring people to stay at home and forego social pleasures bore down heavily on particular groups such as the young, for whom risk taking can be more acceptable than it is for others, especially older people.

In reality it is possible to frame the dilemma in such a way as to try and 'satisfice' each demographic group by managing risks in such a way as to aim for harm reduction. Investment in public health can be seen as investment in protecting a vibrant economy.

In a vibrant democracy the protection of public health should be seen as one of the foundations of individual freedom.

APHORISM 15: GO TO THE PEOPLE

Go to the people, live among them, start
with what they know.

JECH, August 2002, 56: 561

FOR DISCUSSION

+ What are the advantages and disadvantages of a top-down versus a bottom-up approach to protecting and improving health?
+ Under what circumstances is it justifiable to adopt a top-down approach to health protection and improvement?
+ Using the example of the Covid-19 pandemic, illustrate when it was appropriate for governments to be top-down in their approaches and when it was more productive to adopt a bottom-up approach.

CASE STUDY

The community development approach to change is applicable not only to villages and urban slums but also to groups of professional workers in bureaucracies and health care facilities. The notion of sustaining change as part of communities owning the change process is well captured in an anonymous Chinese poem.

Go to the people
Live among them
Start with what they know
Build on what they have
But of the best leaders
When their task is accomplished
Their work done
The people will remark
We have done it ourselves.

There are times, such as during public health emergencies, when it is necessary for governments to take charge and override the levels of public engagement that might be expected during normal times. Nevertheless a prerequisite for the successful handling of public health emergencies is the maintenance of trust between the governed and the governing.

At the heart of maintaining trust is a commitment to openness, transparency and the truth. A well-thought-through approach to public communications fronted up by familiar faces and voices makes this more achievable.

In the UK during the Covid-19 pandemic, the communications strategy was poor. With a government slow to act and running constantly to catch up there was a confusion of messengers and messages, a failure to make optimal use of trusted local Directors of Public Health, and a default position of political campaigning slogans rather than public information based on full disclosure of the facts. The consequences as the emergency unfolded were a progressive loss of trust by the public with an increasing unwillingness to own the measures that were put in place to contain the virus (Ashton, 2020).

APHORISM 16: CONSPIRACIES AGAINST THE LAITY

All professions are conspiracies against the laity.

(Shaw, 1906)
JECH, March 2003, 57: 161

FOR DISCUSSION

✚ What are the main characteristics of professions and those who describe themselves as professionals? How do these differ from trades or crafts?

✚ How does the practice of a health professional focusing on an individual or family member differ from that of a public health professional?

✚ How may the tensions between individual clinical and population level interventions be reconciled?

CASE STUDY

It is a cliché that prostitution is the oldest profession and medicine the second-oldest. In reality prostitution is probably best described as a trade, as normally it lacks the characteristics that are to be found in medicine and other areas of human endeavour that aspire to professional status.

These characteristics include a basis in specialised and theoretical knowledge and practice that enables their practitioners to adapt to changing challenges; an underpinning by institutional arrangements that seek to guarantee to the patient or end user competence based on an ethical framework of practice with appropriate redress if necessary; and legal provision that permits the professional to practise independently but with sanctions that can be imposed should they not live up to the required standards (Friedson, 1970).

These specific features distinguish professions from the trades or crafts from which they have generally evolved. This transition has usually come via organisational forms including guilds set up to protect the livelihoods of those with skill sets that could be differentiated from the range of routine tasks from earlier peasant society. In recent years the so-called 'oldest profession' itself has shown signs of movement along this trajectory with its acceptance in some progressive countries as a legitimate career option complete with state tax and benefit consequences and, in England, the English Collective of Prostitutes can be seen as a concrete manifestation of the beginnings of guild formation en route to professionalisation.

Once professions have become established, the way in which their professionals acquire prestige, wealth and influence is by taking unto themselves a body of knowledge and expertise and only relinquishing it partially in exchange for payment. By not sharing all their acquired knowledge the creation of dependency becomes an important part of this process. Those who can become associated with high-status members of society, such as royalty or celebrities, or by association with high-status institutions, such as teaching hospitals in the nation's capital city, are well-placed to flourish.

But while a doctor may owe an obligation only to the patient in front of them, and possibly the patient's family, in public health that responsibility goes much wider.

Public health, with its focus on protecting and improving the health of whole populations, should share with the more enlightened forms of psychotherapy the desire that individuals and communities should attain, maintain or develop resilience, self-sufficiency and sustainability. It follows that accountability for population health must be via some form of governance arrangement that is congruent with that of the state in which the professional is practising, whether democratic or otherwise. It should be borne in mind that the ethical customs and practices date back to Hippocrates and the Hippocratic Oath, which applies to doctors, whether practising as clinicians or in public health; public health professionals from backgrounds other than medicine are ethically bound by the same tenets.

When it comes to the balance of power and authority between a professional and a member of the public the term *empowerment* currently enjoys popular currency, representing a departure from the recent power imbalance between, for example, doctor and patient, especially in publicly provided health services.

However, this idea of empowerment itself can be patronising if the natural state of grace for individuals is the achievement of mastery over the environment. Striking a style of practice that is respectful of people's gifts and strengths that they bring to problem-solving is the challenge for all public health practitioners and systems; expertise, not necessarily experts!

APHORISM 17: WE'RE DOING IT ALREADY

We're doing it already.

JECH, September 2002, 56: 642

FOR DISCUSSION

+ What experience have you had of trying to achieve change only to be met by 'We're doing it already'?
+ Why do you think people claim that they are 'doing it already' when it seems apparent that they are not?
+ What strategies might you adopt to innovate in the face of opposition?

CASE STUDY

This is a very bad prognostic sign. When change is needed, those who have been responsible for presiding over stagnation inevitably respond to outside scrutiny by claiming to be doing it already, often with a fall-back position of 'It won't work here' (see Aphorism 12).

This defensive response can be infuriating. It is also a warning that what may be needed is subtlety, maturity and a willingness to let other people, no matter how unamenable, take the credit for change and creativity when they have spent many years resisting it. It really is one of the most difficult challenges in public health.

A relevant supplementary aphorism here is that 'It is easier to change your own behaviour than to change somebody else's'. Modelling the desired behaviour through a combination of 'head, heart and hand' (evidence, empathy and non-threatening mentoring) is the route to the soul of change, rather than external judgemental intervention.

We need to give more attention to what lies behind the claim to be 'doing it already'. It may be that in their younger days they were indeed pioneers and that at this stage they object to the implication that their life's work may have been on the wrong track. Reframing the issue as one of a refreshed legacy for those who come after may be the way forward, remembering also the aphorism that allows others to take credit for the innovation (see Aphorism 15).

APHORISM 18: PROPHETS ARE NEVER RECOGNISED IN THEIR OWN COUNTRY

Prophets are never recognised in their own country.

JECH, June 2002, 56: 401

FOR DISCUSSION

✚ What examples do you know of where secular prophets have been ignored in their own place and it has taken an outsider to achieve change?
✚ What do you think lies behind this phenomenon?
✚ What tactics might you deploy to overcome resistance to suggestions for change coming from an insider?

CASE STUDY

The origin of this expression lies in the New Testament of the Christian Bible as reported in the books of the disciples of Jesus. When Jesus began his ministry, he moved from his home town of Nazareth to Capernaum on the coast. Later, having established a reputation as a prophet and a preacher, he returned to Nazareth where he was met with scepticism by those who remembered him as the son of a carpenter. Those who had grown up with him doubted his newly acclaimed abilities and could not accept the claims that were now being made for his wisdom.

It seems that while prophets may not be recognised in their own country, an expert may be regarded as somebody who travels a long distance and brings their own PowerPoint. In the world of medicine, this phenomenon can be seen in the pilgrimages made to study at the feet of renowned medical teachers such as Sigmund Freud in Vienna or to spend time at a prestigious institution such as Yale School of Public Health, the Liverpool or London Schools of Hygiene and Tropical Medicine, or Johns Hopkins in Baltimore (a phenomenon known in medical circles as having got your 'BTA' – 'Been To America').

The process of achieving change is complex and often local institutions and key players are resistant to ideas generated locally. The creative use of facilitation by visitors from abroad can sometimes do the trick; however, see Aphorism 12, 'Not invented here'.

APHORISM 19: PROFESSIONALS SHOULD BE ON TAP, NOT ON TOP

Professionals should be on tap, not on top.

JECH, February 2003, 57: 82

FOR DISCUSSION

+ Can you remember an experience of being patronised by a health professional?
+ What reasons do you think there may be for an imbalance in the power relationship between a health professional and a lay member of the public?
+ How may we redefine the relationship between professionals and lay members of the public to be one of co-production based on equality of purpose?

CASE STUDY

The idea that the relationship between professional workers and communities and citizens should be one of equality is recent and remains novel to many in health care. The Eldon Street Community Association in Liverpool, UK, can trace its roots to the refugees from the Irish potato famine of the 1840s; for more than 170 years they endured the worst health statistics in what was the most important port in the British Empire.

The worm finally turned in the 1970s when the city council decided to forcibly remove the remaining inhabitants from degraded housing conditions. The community organised itself, fought back and reached new heights of self-determination wherein professionals from a range of disciplines were only allowed access to partnership on democratic terms. For too long the community had felt exploited and abused by professionals who came in and stayed long enough to achieve the necessary experience for a career move, while being paid handsomely and usually leaving little enduring contribution.

In the ensuing decades, this community has taken charge of its own housing, employment prospects, education and training, environment, recreation and health, and social care. This shift in power towards co-production based on autonomy was achieved through the development of empathetic understanding between the two parties grounded in the passion of the community, a willingness of professionals to 'listen to the people' and the mobilisation of the community's gifts and talents (McBane, 2008; McKnight, 1995).

APHORISM 20: *PRIMUM NON NOCERE*

Primum non nocere (At least do no harm).

JECH, November 2004, 58: 886

FOR DISCUSSION

+ What examples can you give where intervention was more detrimental than letting sleeping dogs lie?
+ Why do you think that professionals and tradespeople should be inclined to action rather than masterly inactivity where this may be more appropriate?
+ How might we ensure that interventions are only embarked on when they are more likely to result in benefit than harm?

CASE STUDY

From the earliest times, medical students have learnt that the fundamental principle of medical treatment and care is to do no harm. The notion of 'non-maleficence' is one of the principal tenets of bioethics. Despite this, iatrogenic (medically induced) conditions have reached epidemic proportions in many parts of the world.

The application of the precautionary principle to public health has been less clearly enunciated, but it is at least equally relevant. Whether we are talking about interventions at the population, area or group level, or our overarching relationship to Planet Earth, this principle should frame all policy and action.

Inappropriate interventions at a population level are especially likely to occur when they are done *to* a community rather than *with* them. There are many well-meaning examples of attempts to improve the conditions of slum dwellers around the world which have failed to make a difference because they were not carried out in genuine partnership with those affected.

During the Covid-19 pandemic in the UK, a combination of a lack of openness and transparency with the public, manipulation of data and the failure of significant figures to set an example led to a breakdown of trust and an unwillingness of some groups to adhere to safe practices such as mask-wearing and social distancing (Ashton, 2020).

Global warming and massive system disturbance are the realities for public health in the twenty-first century. Unless we become much more committed to taking the precautionary principle seriously and implementing the necessary changes in the way we live, equally across society, then there may be no public health task left to do. The human species may no longer be here (WCED, 1987).

SECTION 3
GETTING STARTED

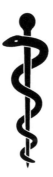

APHORISM 21: LESS IS USUALLY MORE

Less is usually more.

JECH, April 2005, 59: 264

FOR DISCUSSION

+ What do you understand by the idea that less may be more? Can you give an example from everyday life?
+ In efforts to protect and improve health, where do the stereotypes of excessive intervention come from?
+ How might we achieve a better balance between intervention, masterly inactivity and strength-based approaches to health protection and improvement?

CASE STUDY

It is a cliché that physicians prescribe, surgeons cut and psychiatrists answer every question with a question. One of the temptations of professional practice is falling into the trap of thinking that if you *can* do something then you *should*. Individuals and communities that are not functioning well expend considerable amounts of energy on dealing with the consequences. The default position of professionals is too often driven by a desire to intervene instrumentally and to 'fix' problems on their behalf when the solutions may well be found within. Mobilising the intrinsic gifts and assets requires a different approach that has more in common with kung fu and the martial arts, redirecting energy towards more productive ends.

One of the fathers of Asset-Based Community Development, John McKnight, tells us that *'we don't go to the shop before we have seen what we have in the larder or the backyard'*. All individuals should be seen as being half-full rather than half-empty. The art of professional practice is to facilitate co-production through the mobilisation of individual and community assets, only making direct inputs on the basis of a comprehensive mapping of assets and the identification of areas where a unique professional contribution may be appropriate.

Faced with the devastating news that the city council intended to demolish the remaining slum housing in the Vauxhall area of Liverpool and rehouse the residents some distance from their community, the parish priest convened a public meeting. Having brought everybody together to consider their response, he stood back. The community took charge of its own destiny, pushed back against a paternalistic authority and over a period of time regenerated the area on the basis of co-operative housing that met their aspirations.

Public health and other professionals must learn to become minimalists: less is usually more. What is needed in public health is the least intervention that makes the biggest difference. The search for turning points, or turn keys, should inform our efforts to mobilise resources and assets for health.

APHORISM 22: STARTING WHERE THEY ARE

Starting were they are is the key
to providing for underserved groups.

JECH, January 2007, 61: 27

FOR DISCUSSION

+ From your own experience, when are people most likely to follow directions?
+ What are the factors that get in the way of people doing what is in their own best interests?
+ How might professionals best get alongside people from marginalised and underserved groups in order to protect and improve their health and well-being?

CASE STUDY

'*Make contact, maintain contact, make changes*' was the principle behind the first large-scale syringe exchange programme developed for intravenous drug users in Liverpool in 1986. Unless you are in contact with groups whose behaviour is problematic you can do nothing about it. This means that services have to be open-access, non-judgemental, and consumer-friendly.

Maintaining contact is the key to a therapeutic relationship in which changes can be made when the client is ready. The harm reduction approach to drug and sexual health issues has often been resisted by those whose style is paternalistic.

Public health professionals should remember Lowell's aphorism that sometimes it is necessary to forget your principles and do the right thing. The harm reduction approach in Liverpool essentially kept the human immunodeficiency virus (HIV) out of the drug-injecting population. Applied to the vexed issue of teenage pregnancy it led to substantial reductions in pregnancy rates.

APHORISM 23: *CAVEAT EMPTOR*

Caveat emptor (buyer beware) is a warning to consultants: the problem presented is not the real problem.

JECH, March 2007, 61: 220

FOR DISCUSSION

+ What has been your experience of people presenting an issue to you which is not the real issue affecting them?
+ How might you create the conditions under which you may be privy to the real issues underlying a presenting appearance?

CASE STUDY

In borrowing this aphorism from the world of consumerism, Lowell throws us a ball from left field. In a clinical setting we may be familiar with the phenomenon of a patient, who, on the way out says as an apparent afterthought '*by the way, doctor*' and then reveals the real reason for the consultation.

The idea of 'buyer beware' in public health may carry something of the same subtext: in dependency situations the colonially dominated group will tell the more powerful what they want to hear. The art of real empowerment is to get behind the submission by building trust and creating a relationship in which self-esteem is not further damaged or shame becomes collateral damage.

By taking a community's concerns seriously and at face value an entry point is created into understanding the full story and the upstream issues that are the determinants of downstream distress. Many of the downstream manifestations of public health distress are the end result of determinants that may be lost in the stresses of everyday life. (See also Aphorism 11, 'A fish is the last one to see the water'.) Alcohol and drug abuse, teenage pregnancy, violence and self-harm are among the everyday harms that result from deprivation and disadvantage, discrimination and the resulting lack of control, sense of coherence and poor esteem (Durkheim, 1975; Antonovsky, 1987; Mental Health Foundation, 2016).

APHORISM 24: DON'T FOLLOW THE YELLOW BRICK ROAD

Don't follow the yellow brick road.
(If you always do what you always did you will always get what you always got.)

JECH, May 2006, 60: 447

FOR DISCUSSION

✚ What was the significance of the yellow brick road in the film *The Wizard of Oz*?

✚ Why should we be wary of assuming that a yellow brick road is the path to success in public health?

✚ What are the implications of following the yellow brick road?

CASE STUDY

In the novel *The Wonderful Wizard of Oz*, a road paved with yellow bricks leads to the Emerald City, the imperial capital of the land of Oz (Baum, 1900). The novel's heroine, Dorothy, sets off down the road in search of the Wizard rumoured to be found there, experiencing many diversions and adventures on the way.

The nature of public health is such that the challenges are constantly changing and that although core principles can be identified, the same solutions will not necessarily achieve the same results. Old problems disappear or reappear in a different form and new ones come along.

The Victorian agenda of poor sanitation, polluted drinking water, adulterated and unsafe food, air pollution and cheap gin has been succeeded by new variants on the same themes. Because of the time dimension, history is not a pendulum but a helix and we must constantly adapt our responses even when problems look similar. It is rare to find a direct pathway between intervention and result and often a whole systems approach is needed to tackle the upstream determinants of ill health. Often it is necessary to take a leaf out of the sailors' navigation guide and to 'tack' our way towards the desired destination.

Einstein is reputed to have said that the definition of insanity is '*doing the same thing over and over and expecting different results*' (Wilczek, 2015). Following the 'beaten path' in public health without questioning, without critique, is a dangerous strategy. Just ask a lemming. If you always do what you always did you will always get what you always got. Every organisation is perfectly designed to get the results that it achieves.

———————————————————

APHORISM 25: COMMUNITY ORGANISERS BEWARE

Community organisers beware: there is no such thing as an unorganised community.

JECH, April 2006, 60: 284

FOR DISCUSSION

✚ Consider a community with which you are most familiar. What do you see as its strengths and weaknesses?

✚ Can you think of any community you know which has no strengths? Can you think of any community which has no weaknesses?

✚ How might professionals best approach work with communities so as to play to their strengths and not exacerbate their weaknesses?

CASE STUDY

No matter how disadvantaged, all communities are to a greater or lesser extent self-organising. Just as nature abhors a vacuum, so the instinct for coherence runs deep and social stratification and order usually emerge even in the most desperate situations. While in earlier times forms of community development associated with traditional and colonial society were paternalistic, more recently strength-based approaches to community organisation have come to the fore.

Asset-Based Community Development (ABCD), which is associated with the work of John McKnight and his colleagues in Chicago, sees communities as being half-full rather than half-empty. By a process of mapping the human and environmental assets of neighbourhoods and communities, ABCD facilitates their mobilisation towards community-derived goals through the agency of community organisers or 'gappers'. Gappers are the connecting lubricant between associations of groups of citizens, the resources that are to be found among and around them and the institutions with their bureaucrats and professionals who may be able to unlock access to the institutional resources that are under their control. In his early life a young Barack Obama trained as a community organiser with the ABCD team in Chicago (Kretzmann and McKnight, 1993; McKnight and Block, 2010).

The challenge for professionals and bureaucracies is to reorientate their mode of practice towards ABCD in which they are 'on tap, not on top'.

APHORISM 26: SELF-FULFILLING PROPHECY KILLS

Self-fulfilling prophecy kills.

JECH, 2006, 60: 570

FOR DISCUSSION

+ What different types of evidence are available to the public health practitioner?
+ What is the difference between prophecy, projection and prediction?
+ Does prophecy have any part to play in public health?

CASE STUDY

Prophecy involves predicting what will happen in the future on the basis of some form of divine inspiration or inner voice. In the absence of objective evidence it is at the opposite end of a spectrum running through projection to prediction. While projection involves a rational estimate derived from extrapolations based on current trends, prediction is a form of forecasting which is often, but not always, based on experience or conventional scientific knowledge; it may involve triangulation with a variety of inputs including the lived experience of ordinary people.

In the sense that pure prophecy depends on insights that are not available to third parties, it may take us into dangerous territory. If it is based on the accumulation of wisdom from previous experience perhaps it merits a voice at the table; however, one of the most dangerous conditions for community health is indifference to the status quo or the belief that you can't beat the system. Talk about self-fulfilling prophecies!

Scepticism about the value of masks and face coverings as a defence against coronavirus was probably responsible for many thousands of avoidable deaths during the Covid-19 pandemic.

APHORISM 27: COLUMBUS ON THE NEED FOR STRATEGY

Columbus on the need for strategy.

JECH, April 2003, 57: 235

FOR DISCUSSION

✚ What are the main elements of a strategic way of thinking?
✚ What is the main danger of not having a strategic approach to public health?
✚ How might the imperatives of today be met without compromising our ability to anticipate and prevent the threats of tomorrow?

CASE STUDY

Strategy is about the long term and having clear goals to inform daily decisions that will move us in the right direction. Such is the pressure of everyday life and the unexpected events that are constantly cropping up that it is all too easy to become immersed in the daily round to the detriment of longer-term progress.

When Christopher Columbus set sail from Cadiz to America in 1492 he had no idea where he was going. When he got there he had no idea where he was, and when he returned to Spain he had no idea where he had been.

The argument for having a strategy is that if you don't know where you want to go you won't know whether you have achieved your ambitions and you may miss opportunities on the way. A strategy is essential, allied to a practical orientation and a drilling down to the operational level, 'a clean mind and dirty hands'.

The pursuit of a strategy requires capacity- and capability-building and asset mobilisation to support those going where no man or woman has been before.

APHORISM 28: POLITICS IS MEDICINE ON A LARGE SCALE

Medicine is a social science and politics is nothing but medicine on a large scale.

JECH, August 2006, 60: 671

FOR DISCUSSION

✚ Is there such a thing as politics-free public health?

✚ Can you give examples of where the politics of a public health issue assumed a prominence in the public arena?

✚ How might public health professionals best resolve the tensions that exist in practising public health in a political environment?

CASE STUDY

The German cell biologist Rudolf Virchow is credited with the aphorism that *'Medicine is a social science and politics is nothing else but medicine on a large scale'* (Virchow, 1848, quoted in Sigerist, 1941, p 93). Building on the essentially political nature of medicine and public health, it has also been asserted that *'Parliament is the dispensary of public health'*, alluding to the plethora of legal frameworks that underpin the protection of public health and the provision of medical and social care. At the heart of these statements is the distribution of power and influence.

Given our understanding of the nature of the determinants of health and disease, and in particular the gross inequalities that characterise the health of different populations in many countries, it may come as a surprise to some that there should be controversy about the essentially political nature of health (Marmot et al, 2010). In reality there are those who wish to see the practice of medicine and health-related disciplines as purely matters of applied science.

A historical perspective on the reductions in death rates and improvements in well-being over the past 200 years is illuminating in this regard. Most of the progress in these areas predates the advent of scientific medicine and can be accounted for by improvements in living and working conditions, better nutrition brought about by increases in agricultural productivity and cheaper foods, and the adoption of birth control resulting in smaller families enjoying a higher standard of living (McKeown, 1976; Ashton and Seymour, 1989; Ashton, 2019).

———————————————

APHORISM 29: STARTING A RUMOUR

Starting a rumour and spending other people's money.

JECH, August 2003, 57: 615

FOR DISCUSSION

+ When was the last time you started a rumour? Was it something positive that inspired others to become involved?
+ What do you think is the secret to getting others to sign up to your pet ideas?
+ What does public health have up its sleeve that can galvanise others into action if used in the right way?

CASE STUDY

When Columbus discovered America, not only did he have no strategy but he did it with somebody else's money (the Queen of Spain). Bridging the gap between starting a rumour (in the case of Columbus that there was a new world out there somewhere, waiting to be discovered, or in the case of public health that change is possible) and mobilising the resources for change, is at the heart of public health.

How often have you heard somebody say that they can't do anything to improve health without knowing where the money is coming from first? Yet public health is essentially about shaping and influencing the actions and choices of others and other sectors. An effective public health practitioner should be adept at mobilising assets and resources and spending other people's money, but for this to happen on any meaningful scale it is essential for other players involved to feel a sense of ownership.

Violence is ubiquitous in societies around the world and it is often accompanied by a fatalistic attitude that assumes there is little that can be done about it. In recent years it has become apparent that violence is not inevitable and that much can be done to reduce its prevalence. In 2002 the World Health Organization published its seminal *World Report on Violence and Health* (WHO, 2002). This comprehensive review defined and measured the extent of the problem in member states. The report demonstrated that levels of violence fluctuate in time and space and that it is not necessary to accept levels of violence as inevitable. Since then the evidence has accumulated of the effectiveness of interventions beginning from the first 1000 days of life, through childhood and adolescence and into adulthood.

The WHO report drew attention to the essentially orphan status of violence prevention. While police forces and criminal justice systems pick up the pieces from violence in one sense, and hospital casualty departments and social services in another, a comprehensive partnership approach that brings together many agencies is essential if violence is to be prevented. One of the unique contributions to this from public health is the synthesis of action-orientated intelligence.

I have often contended that in public health we need not Directors of Finance but Directors of Resources. The mindset that starts with financial resources in health finishes up with a fixation on doctors and nurses, bricks and mortar and bits of kit. These are important but resources for health run much wider and include many human and environmental assets that lie outside the bailiwick of something called 'health'. Protecting and maintaining health requires widespread expertise at least as much as dedicated 'experts'. Nowhere is this more apparent than in the prevention of violence.

Starting the rumour that violence can be prevented would be a good first step in tackling this ubiquitous problem. Reaching a tipping point in reducing levels of violence requires all the skills of public health in mobilising broad-based partnerships informed by practical intelligence (Gladwell, 2000; Ashton, 2019).

APHORISM 30: EDWIN CHADWICK AND *THE TIMES*

On The Times, Edwin Chadwick,

and the 'nanny state'.

JECH, January 2004, 58: 5

FOR DISCUSSION

+ What do you understand by the idea of the 'nanny state'?
+ When might it be appropriate for governments to intervene directly in the freedoms of the public in the interests of public health?
+ What should the limits of government intervention be?

CASE STUDY

The London *Times* is said to have claimed that it would prefer to take its chance with the cholera *'than be bullied into health by Mr Chadwick'*. Edwin Chadwick was one of the leaders of reform of the Poor Laws in England and a disciple of Jeremy Bentham, whose philosophy of *'The greatest good for the greatest number'* was very influential in the Victorian Poor Law Movement. As author of the *Report on the Sanitary Condition of the Labouring Population of Great Britain*, published in 1842, and later as Commissioner of the General Board of Health from 1848 to its abolition in 1854, Chadwick was a public health advocate who frequently alienated vested interests that resented interference in their freedom of action (Chadwick, 1964 [1842]; Wohl, 1984; Ashton, 2019).

The argument about the appropriate role of the state rumbled on in Europe throughout the nineteenth century: minimalist, only concerned with property rights, or interventionist on behalf of social justice and a phenomenon called society, protector of the weak, the poor, the young, the aged and infirm, giving voice to the underdog.

In recent decades and a contemporary climate of neoliberal economics, the same arguments have been to the fore. We accept that individuals may have no chance alone to deal with bioterrorism and outbreaks of novel viruses such as SARS or Covid-19, or natural disasters, but how much chance do they have when faced with the commercial determinants of ill health – the promotion of tobacco, alcohol, gambling, junk food, or obesogenic personal transport (the motor car)?

The notion of the 'nanny state' clearly has a long pedigree and surfaced again during the Covid-19 pandemic, when the tension between individual freedom and the protection of the vulnerable was played out in real time with often late and inconsistent interventions by government with contradictory messaging.

Where would Edwin Chadwick, who pressed for slum improvement and sanitary reform in his time, stand today? What has the London *Times* to say on such questions?

SECTION 4
MAKING A DIFFERENCE

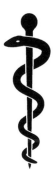

APHORISM 31: THE HALF-LIFE OF EVIDENCE

The half-life of a medical fact is about four and a half years (Lowell S Levin).

JECH, November 2003, 57: 887

FOR DISCUSSION

✚ Where does the generation and testing of hypotheses fit in to the advancement of science?

✚ Can you think of any scientific 'facts' that have changed dramatically in your lifetime?

✚ How can we best respond to the constantly changing scenario of scientific 'facts'?

CASE STUDY

Lowell S Levin was widely read and a fount of wisdom. When he was giving one of his informal seminars such as 'An Evening with Lowell S Levin' he would often drop in a statement such as '*The half-life of a medical fact is four and a half years*' to make a point (rather as in Douglas Adams' novel *The Hitchhiker's Guide to the Galaxy*, in which '42' was the answer to '*life, the universe and everything*'; Adams, 1979).

Lowell reminds us of the dynamic and ephemeral nature of knowledge. More than 17,000 new biomedical books are published every year along with over 30,000 biomedical journals. Knowledge management matters if we are not to drown in the irrelevant.

Science advances by the creation of hypotheses based on the known facts; efforts are then made to disprove a hypothesis and replace it with another. Should the tested hypothesis still stand it becomes that much more secure and lives to be tested again another day.

In recent years, scientific knowledge has accelerated and a commitment to lifelong learning is a prerequisite for professionals to maintain adequate levels of professional practice. When I was a medical student, it was considered that peptic ulcers were caused by an excess of gastric acid in the stomach and treatments, both medical and surgical, included partial or complete removal of the stomach. However, in 1982 it was discovered that both peptic ulcers and gastric cancer were associated with the bacterium *helicobacter pylori*, which could be readily treated with antibiotics.

During the Covid-19 pandemic there was an initial standoff between senior public health advisers who believed that the wearing of masks and face coverings may be of no benefit in controlling the spread of the virus and those who cited their benefit from both historical and contemporary experience in particular from Asia. As the pandemic progressed there was general acceptance that masks and face coverings had an important part to play.

———————————————

APHORISM 32: PROOF AND EVIDENCE

No evidence of proof is not evidence of
no proof.

JECH, February 2007, 61: 134

FOR DISCUSSION

✚ What do you understand as the difference between association and causation?
✚ When it comes to public health, where does the burden of proof lie?
✚ Why might no evidence of proof not be evidence of no proof?

CASE STUDY

Setting aside the plethora of double negatives in the questions under discussion, this issue is an important one. It carries traps that even senior public health advisers can fall into as, for example, in the vexed issue of the value of masks and face coverings in the prevention of the Covid-19 virus.

Unlike in the science laboratory, where it may be possible to hold variables constant while one variable is changed to explore cause and effect, it is different in the world of everyday life. Robert Koch identified four criteria that must be satisfied in order to identify the causative agent in the case of infectious disease but we must be more imaginative when it comes to many of the challenges that confront us in everyday public health where multifactorial determinants are the norm (Barry, 2004).

Koch postulates that:

✚ the micro-organism must be present in all cases of the disease;
✚ the pathogen can be isolated from the diseased host and grown in pure culture;
✚ the pathogen from the pure culture must cause the disease when inoculated into a healthy susceptible laboratory animal;
✚ the pathogen must be re-isolated from the new host and shown to be the same as the originally inoculated pathogen.

Koch's work and his insights led to major breakthroughs in the fields of microbiology and virology, and underpins our knowledge of the influenza virus and most recently the novel coronavirus that causes Covid-19. However, other criteria are necessary when it comes to understanding whether, for example, mask-wearing outside the laboratory confers protection against either the mask-wearer or somebody in close proximity to an infected person.

Causal thinking in the health sciences rests on a set of criteria including the strength and direction of the association between presumed cause and effect, the time sequencing, specificity, consistency, coherence in terms of what is known, and predictive performance (Susser, 1973). In the case of the value of masks in the prevention of coronavirus transmission, laboratory experiments have been of little value in understanding the impact of mask-wearing at a population level, with all its complexities. The lived experience of millions of people in Asian countries during the pandemic came to trump the academic theories of advisers in the West.

In recent times, a series of public health incidents should have alerted us to the importance of not being seduced by reductionist and positivist approaches to science. Both the bovine spongiform encephalopathy (BSE) disaster and the scepticism about the value of wearing masks and face coverings as part of a package of measures to control Covid-19 are stark reminders of the importance of humility and an open mind when it comes to protecting the public's health (Ashton, 2020).

The question of 'on whom should the burden of proof lie one way or the other in contentious situations?' reminds us of the essentially political nature of public health, of the necessity of admitting when knowledge is incomplete and a willingness to shoulder the responsibility of giving advice nevertheless, and taking account of the precautionary principle.

APHORISM 33: THE ART AND SCIENCE
OF PUBLIC HEALTH

Public health is an art but should

also be a science.

JECH, May 2007, 61: 373

FOR DISCUSSION

✚ Which sciences underpin the practice of public health?
✚ In what sense should public health be regarded as an art as well as a science?
✚ How may the tensions inherent in the schism between the arts and the sciences be reconciled in the practice of public health?

CASE STUDY

According to Charles Winslow in his enduring definition:

Public Health is the science and the art of preventing disease, prolonging life, and promoting physical health and efficiency through organized community efforts for the sanitation of the environment, the control of community infections, the education of the individual in principles of personal hygiene, the organization of medical and nursing service for the early diagnosis and preventive treatment of disease, and the development of the social machinery which will ensure to every individual in the community a standard of living adequate for the maintenance of health.

(Winslow, 1920)

While the scientific underpinnings of public health lie in biology, physics and chemistry, they also lie in other fields of scientific endeavour including those of the environment and not least the social sciences of which anthropology is often neglected. Anthropology as the study of how human groups live and what it is that makes us human is the bridge into the humanities and the arts.

In his 1959 Rede Lecture, C P Snow explored the schism between the humanities and the sciences which is a fracture line in our understanding of ourselves and how we live (Snow, 1959). Failure to address this can lead to major errors in public health. During the Ebola epidemic in West Africa in 2014, medical and biological scientists quickly identified the virus responsible together with the vulnerability of those in most intimate contact with the victims. These included, especially, health care workers and the family members responsible for the ritual bathing of the dead. However, they made the error of assuming that those who needed to be influenced to change the ritual practices were the male village chiefs. It was only when anthropologists became involved that it became clear that it was the village women's committees who held sway over such matters. Understanding the lived experience of ordinary people is a vital component of effective public health.

Historically in many countries public health was led by male doctors and engineers. Since the advent of the New Public Health in the 1970s it has embraced the qualitative as well as the quantitative sciences, gender parity and a multidisciplinary approach (Ashton and Seymour, 1989; Ashton, 2019).

APHORISM 34: ON STRATEGIC UNDERVIEW

The need for strategic underview.

JECH, October 2003, 57: 808

FOR DISCUSSION

✚ What do you think might be meant by the concept of a strategic underview?
✚ Why do you think an underview might be as important as an overview?
✚ How might you ensure that those responsible for strategy kept their feet on the ground?

CASE STUDY

Top-down, bottom-up, there is a great deal of discussion about how to modernise and achieve change, particularly in public services. We have been inching our way from feudal organisational forms through the free market and paternalistic organisations.

The current received wisdom is about the need to empower frontline staff and to shift the balance of power away from the centre towards the periphery. Decentralisation and participation are key words. The catastrophic failure of over-centralisation of measures to test and trace for the coronavirus has been starkly exposed during the Covid-19 pandemic in the UK.

More generally there is often talk, rather like sheep and goats, of people who are either 'strategic' (visionaries, leaders, highly paid people) or 'operational' (the people who do the work at the sharp end and are much lower paid with much less job security, and who are sacrificed when things go wrong). The crucial importance of frontline operatives in hospitals, care homes and essential public service work has been highlighted during the pandemic, when many have paid the ultimate price and died from viral infection while saving the lives of others or keeping the economy moving.

There is a story about President Kennedy visiting the space centre at Cape Canaveral; when he asked a cleaner what his job was, the cleaner is said to have replied that he was helping to put a man on the moon.

In Liverpool in the 1980s, when teenage pregnancy was a hot issue, a proposal was put to the Health Authority to reinvest family planning money in street-level sexual health services for young people. One morning the chairman of the Health Authority came into the office with an announcement to make. The previous evening he had arrived unannounced at just such a clinic and mingled with the young women clients who were queuing on the pavement, many of them with their boyfriends. He signed off the proposal with enthusiasm.

The reality is that, in life, we need a whole systems approach, where we acknowledge and respect our interdependence. This means that not only should the high-flying leaders keep their feet on the ground, while maintaining their eyes above the horizon, but that the 'doers' should understand how their tasks, so often considered modest, contribute to major strategic achievements: the need for strategic underview.

APHORISM 35: THE HIDDEN HEALTH CARE SYSTEM

The hidden health care system.

JECH, November 2005, 59: 933

FOR DISCUSSION

✦ What do you understand by 'the hidden health care system'?
✦ What do you think is the ratio between formal and informal health care in everyday life?
✦ How might we optimise the balance between informal and formal health care and by so doing improve population health?

CASE STUDY

There is a hidden health care system with clear definitions and roles. Lowell S Levin studied and wrote about this phenomenon throughout his long career in public health and claimed that over 80 per cent of health care takes place in a big pool without the 'benefit' of 'medical clergy' (Levin and Adler, 1981). In traditional societies the caring roles have often fallen to women, but this is slowly changing.

Lowell's contributions formed part of a critique of mainstream medical practice which included that by Ivan Illich, whose book *Medical Nemesis*, published in 1974, argued that the medical establishment had become a major threat to health (Illich, 1974). Illich was an early collaborator of John McKnight, one of the founders of Asset-Based Community Development (McKnight and Block, 2010).

At the heart of Asset-Based Community Development is the recognition that human communities possess a wide range of skills that pre-date the commodification and division of roles that grew out of the industrial revolution; and that underneath the surface most individuals and communities are half full rather than half empty. Mapping and mobilising the gifts and assets of communities is seen as the route to an abundant life.

If you consider, even for somebody with a long-term condition such as type II diabetes, how much contact time in hours they might expect to have with a health professional during the course of a year it becomes obvious that they, themselves, are the frontline of medical care together with their significant others and must become 'expert patients'. This should start in the home and school with support for the self-management of common conditions rather than by recourse to experts (see Aphorism 16, 'Conspiracies against the laity').

Embracing an Asset-Based Approach to Community Organisation and Development is challenging both to businesses that have been based on making traditional domestic activities into commodities that can be bought and sold and to organised labour that has come to expect that the public will pay for activities that they could well carry out for themselves with resulting satisfaction and material benefit. It is likely that from the ensuing tension will emerge new forms of economic activity and that this will be reinforced by the reappraisal of work-life balance that is taking place as a result of the Covid-19 pandemic.

On the broader canvas, the professionalisation of everyday life can be illustrated by the development of the highly lucrative funeral business from what was once a community activity. My auntie Marj was a nurse in Lancashire in the years after the Second World War when it was still common in rural areas for a local nurse, like her, to lay out bodies in the front parlour of a neighbour's house. She was an asset to her community, carrying out a function which has now been largely commodified and professionalised.

William Morris' definition of health (Aphorism 8) anticipated the reappraisal of life in which a holistic vision replaced the soul-destroying cycle of industrialised working 'deprived of all enjoyment of the natural beauty of the world' and amusements 'to quicken the flow of their spirits from time to time'.

APHORISM 36: BE CAREFUL WHAT YOU ARE SELLING

Be careful what you are selling, medical care
is the third cause of death (Lowell S Levin).

JECH, March 2005, 59: 181

FOR DISCUSSION

+ What are the most common risks to health in everyday life?
+ What do you understand by iatrogenesis?
+ How might we best move towards a situation in which medical risks are reduced and co-production becomes a meaningful goal?

CASE STUDY

Everyday life can be hazardous, especially in the early years when environmental hazards account for a large proportion of premature death and ill health. In the later years, falls become a danger with increasing frailty and may mark the beginning of terminal decline.

Self-harm and injury from violence are features of early adult life, with suicide becoming a particular phenomenon of men entering middle age; homicide risk varies by gender, with the home being the most dangerous place for a woman and the street for a man. However, medical care begins to become problematic as we age and accumulate long-term conditions with the increasing prospect of multiple pharmacological and surgical treatments.

This aphorism is self-explanatory and the iatrogenic side effects of medical care are significant contributors to morbidity and mortality. However, there is often a touching belief in the efficacy of medical care that is shared by professionals and the public. We must constantly question where the most appropriate intervention points are to improve and protect the public's health and not be seduced uncritically by interventions for their own sake. Openness and transparency are the keys to shared responsibility and improved outcomes with an emphasis on evidence-based practice, clinical audit and blame-free learning. There should only be witch hunts when there are witches.

In the age of the internet, medical knowledge has been democratised and it is common for patients to consult their medical advisers already equipped with knowledge about their ailments and the pros and cons of treatment.

In his report *An Organisation with a Memory*, the Chief Medical Officer for England, Sir Liam Donaldson, made the case for openness and transparency coupled with a no blame culture in publishing outcome data for medical interventions (Donaldson, 2002). Drawing on examples of quality improvement from the airline industry, Donaldson argued that health workers should adopt a non-hierarchical approach to learning from near misses in clinical settings.

APHORISM 37: THE CONSPIRACY OF SILENCE

The conspiracy of silence in health care and its hazards.

JECH, November 2006, 60: 913

FOR DISCUSSION

+ Why do you think there is a reluctance to be open with the public about errors in medicine and health care?
+ What approach is most likely to do away with the conspiracy of silence?
+ What are the obstacles that will need to be overcome?

CASE STUDY

Doctors and other health care workers enjoy high levels of trust among the general public. Despite the ancient edict of '*Primum non nocere*', errors of omission and of commission do occur in hospitals, clinics and the community.

Every year many thousands of people die or suffer serious long-term medical injury as a result of the most basic failures of procedure and sometimes because of the criminal intent of professionals (see Aphorism 36, 'Be careful what you are selling'). There is a conspiracy of silence about the quality of medical care and its hazards.

In his report *An Organisation with a Memory*, former United Kingdom Chief Medical Officer Sir Liam Donaldson described how a systematic approach to reducing medical harm could be adopted based on the experiences of the airline industry (Donaldson, 2002). In the airline industry the creation of open feedback that dispensed with the intimidating impact of hierarchy on the flight deck led to much improved aviation safety.

In recent years there have been many incidents of serious clinical service failure in the United Kingdom where such an approach may have prevented dire consequences for patients and their families. These have included scandals at Alder Hey Children's Hospital in Liverpool, Stafford Hospital and the University Hospitals of Morecambe Bay NHS Foundation Trust (Ashton, 2019).

On 31 January 2000, British general practitioner Harold Shipman was found guilty of the murder of 15 patients under his care with estimates that he may have killed as many as 250. A retrospective analysis of his practice population found a statistical excess of deaths. Nor is the private sector exempt from this kind of scandal, with many health care workers dismissed from the National Health Service subsequently finding employment in private practice.

These disasters can only be addressed through joint professional and consumer action in a genuine partnership: the hammer and the anvil, or, as the South Africans say '*one hand washes the other*'. The implication of this is much more openness about results, outcomes and failings and a willingness for professionals to be self-critical and for the public to be forgiving.

APHORISM 38: ACHIEVING CHANGE

Achieving change is about more than ticking boxes.

JECH, February 2004, 58: 102

FOR DISCUSSION

✚ In a democracy, what are the prerequisites for achieving change in professional practice?

✚ In recent years, regular professional appraisal has become an integral part of routine professional life. What are the pros and cons?

✚ Can you give examples of where public health practice has been changed for the better?

CASE STUDY

The argument about the value of targets in improving performance arouses strong emotions. We know that the battle for hearts and minds, for buy-in and ownership, are at least as important as the accountancy-driven approach to improved performance epitomised by the schoolmaster Gradgrind in Charles Dickens' novel *Hard Times*, who knew the price of everything and the value of nothing. Presentation and packaging need to be more than skin deep.

The adoption of annual professional appraisal can be a mixed blessing, especially if it is used as a method of performance management rather than in support of professional development. In the former case the potential loss of trust risks losing the personal ownership of innovation and quality improvement which should be the goal of appraisal.

Totalitarian states such as the former Soviet Union often pursue top-down performance management with a plethora of five-year plans and goals which become a meaningless distraction and can lead to gaming and box-ticking. An empowered workforce will be looking to innovate and improve practice because of the sense of satisfaction it can bring.

In the United Kingdom during the first months of the 2020 Covid-19 pandemic there were almost daily pronouncements by ministers of the numbers of Covid-19 tests that were to be reached within days or weeks. It soon became apparent that the numbers involved were a charade resulting in a loss of public trust that probably contributed to the weakening of adherence to virus control measures such as mask-wearing and social distancing (Ashton, 2020).

When I was a student at Newcastle medical school in the 1960s we used to retreat from the anatomy dissecting room into the bowels of the basement in search of coffee and sustenance from a distant outreach of the Students' Union Refectory. All that was on offer was beans on toast and poor quality tea and coffee. Protests to the head of catering in the Students' Union produced a positive response, soon to be followed by a new menu posted on the wall beside the coffee counter – but still, all you could get was beans on toast and poor quality tea and coffee.

APHORISM 39: LET THE DOUGH RISE SLOWLY

In public health let the dough rise slowly
(but not too slowly) (forced rhubarb).

JECH, April 2007, 61: 281

FOR DISCUSSION

✚ Can you think of an example of where the pressure to deliver quickly has led to a poor result?
✚ How can you best manage the tension between pressure for delivery and ensuring that the outcome is the best it can be?

CASE STUDY

Being effective in public health is demanding and requires a complex skill set: curiosity, an ability to listen and observe, to reflect back and to constantly learn; to analyse and report; to think on your feet; to communicate well with many different types of audience, the mainstream and social media; 'to fill a room'; and to have a clean mind and dirty hands.

Whilst decisive and effective action is called for in public health emergencies, in other situations there may be a temptation to intervene inappropriately when it may be better for a community to find its own solutions through self-organisation. Judicious intervention comes with experience, perhaps, with some offline support akin to coaching.

Admitting ignorance is vitally important in avoiding mistakes and, in problem-solving, being distracted can be a good thing. The tendency is to be drawn in to an analytic and reductionist assessment of what we are faced with, when intuition and affective awareness of what is impacting on the community can give real insights into what the real way forward is. Sleep on it, reflect and listen.

During the Covid-19 pandemic, the British government claimed to be '*following the science*' while dismissing evidence of the effectiveness of intervention measures from other countries and expressing false degrees of certainty when it would have been better to admit ignorance. Many lives were lost unnecessarily.

At the same time as claiming to follow the science, the government was claiming to have all the answers and to be in control of the situation when it was clear to many that this was not the case. By putting too much faith in experts and failing to recognise the importance of candid communication and full public engagement, the opportunity to mobilise the capacity and capability of ordinary people as slow burn assets in fighting the pandemic was mostly lost. By infantilising the public with its mixed and political messaging the government alienated people and trust was lost.

When vaccine development reached an advanced stage, the UK and Russian governments embarked on a political race to be the first country to approve vaccines for public use. By jumping the gun, even though the vaccines approved may have been safe, and by not waiting to approve them together in concert with other countries in solidarity, a huge risk was taken of undermining public trust not only in Covid-19 vaccines but in other important vaccine programmes that have been of huge benefit to public health. Forced rhubarb may not be better than that which has been allowed to ripen normally.

How may things have been different if the slow burn had been married to the science?

_____

APHORISM 40: A SENSE OF PLACE

Epidemiology and a sense of place.

JECH, July 2004, 58: 545

FOR DISCUSSION

+ How would you best describe yourself in time, place and person?
+ What have been the most important influences in making you the person you are today?
+ Could you imagine how you might be different if you had grown up in a different place?

CASE STUDY

My books are always about living in places, not just rushing through them. As we get to know Europe slowly, tasting the wines, cheeses and characters of different countries you begin to realise that the determinant of any culture is after all... the spirit of place. Just as one particular vineyard will always give you a special wine with discernible characteristics, so a Spain, an Italy, a Greece will always give you the same type of culture... will express itself through the human beings just as it does through its wild flowers.

(Durrell, 1960)

As one of the major disciplines underpinning the study of public health, epidemiology concerns itself with the analysis of time, place, and person. Durrell's beautiful insight can make our epidemiological teaching seem one dimensional. If we are to unpack the epidemiological study of place we need help from the social sciences, anthropology and, not least, personal narrative and lived experience. We must embrace the interrelationship between humans and environment which is our habitat.

One of the most dangerous traps for the public health professional is to see the world only through their own eyes and their own background. To be able to walk in another person's shoes is the beginning of empathy and understanding.

During the 2014 Ebola epidemic in West Africa the failure of outside advisers to understand that it was the women's committees that held sway over ritual burial practices led to a delay in bringing the disease under control and to unnecessary deaths.

The World Health Organization Healthy Cities Project that began in 1986 is now a global programme including thousands of cities worldwide. The project focuses on the cities, towns and villages which shape the lives of their residents where they '*live, love, work and play*' (Ashton, 2019). While all cities share a set of challenges in protecting and providing for their citizens, each is in its own way unique as a place '*to grow people in*'.

SECTION 5
REFLECTIONS

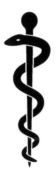

APHORISM 41: PUBLIC HEALTH IS AN INVESTMENT

Public health is an investment, not a cost.

JECH, March 2006, 60: 212

FOR DISCUSSION

✦ What are the arguments for and against public health being seen primarily as a cost rather than an investment?

✦ Why do you think that this is an argument that just won't go away?

✦ Can you give an example of when these arguments became very heated in the public domain?

CASE STUDY

The globally dominant economic model, has, until recently, been one based on the extraction and exploitation of human and environmental resources with little attention being paid to resilience and sustainability. This has begun to change, especially since the World Commission on Environment and Development's publication of *Our Common Future* in 1987 and the adoption of the Sustainable Development Goals by the United Nations in 2015, but became highly contentious during the Covid-19 pandemic in 2020 (WCED, 1987; United Nations, 2015).

During the Covid-19 pandemic, the health and well-being of the public, especially that of older and more vulnerable people, was set in opposition to the economy by some politicians and commentators. At the height of the pandemic, ethical principles were breached in that guidelines were issued by the National Institute for Health and Care Excellence that seemed to recommend that Covid-19 sufferers who were frail or who had long-term conditions including autism should not be considered for intensive hospital treatment (Iacobucci, 2020).

Notwithstanding such important ethical considerations, there was a failure to appreciate the interdependence of the economy and public health and well-being. Those countries that acted decisively and early in the pandemic, such as China, Taiwan, South Korea, New Zealand and the Scandinavian countries with the exception of Sweden, experienced less economic harm and a quicker economic rebound than those that had neglected their public health systems and failed to prioritise active public health interventions early in the crisis.

In the future, public health action will need to be looked on to a large extent as an investment comparable to financial investment. Health investment analysts will need to develop skills in mediation, arbitration and negotiation to ensure that health outcomes are optimised from a wide range of investment perspectives – governmental, private and communal. These investments in such areas as housing, transport, agriculture, energy, culture, media and sport mean that the days of looking on public health as a cost are limited.

APHORISM 42: WILLIAM HENRY DUNCAN'S ESTABLISHMENT

The following is my entire establishment

– your servant, William Henry Duncan

JECH, August 2004, 58: 717

FOR DISCUSSION

+ What are the resources available to public health?
+ How may an asset-based approach to public health be developed?
+ What are the obstacles to seeing resources for health as being about more than dedicated personnel and budgets?

CASE STUDY

How often do we hear public health practitioners claiming that they cannot do what is needed without more dedicated resources, and how often are they told that public health systems can only cope with three or four priorities? To which my answer is '*Which of the biblical ten commandments is optional?*'

When the country's first Medical Officer of Health, William Henry Duncan, set about his pioneering work in Liverpool in the 1840s and 1850s it must have seemed that he would be overwhelmed by the cholera and the slum conditions. The city had grown rapidly from a small fishing village to become a major port in the British Empire and as a consequence was beset with slums and disease. Duncan had been working as a general practitioner in the central area of the city in the 1830s and became so concerned about the living conditions that he carried out a survey that became the basis of a report to Edwin Chadwick, who was conducting an enquiry into the operation of the Poor Law (Ashton and Seymour, 1989).

Duncan's work as an early public health doctor, researcher and advocate was to lead to his appointment as Medical Officer of Health in 1847 and together with the borough engineer James Newlands and sanitary inspector Thomas Fresh he was able to head off the worst impact of the 1849 pandemic of Asian cholera which arrived in the city at the same time as 300,000 starving migrants had arrived from Ireland, escaping the potato famine there (Frazer, 1947).

When Edwin Chadwick had written to Duncan enquiring as to his establishment as Medical Officer of Health, Duncan's response was: '*The following is my entire establishment, Your Servant William Henry Duncan.*'

Public health is about mobilising and working through others if it is about anything. Duncan worked with the Health of Towns Association, with its preponderance of participants from the business community, the churches, other civic leaders, and even the occasional other doctor, to mobilise those resources needed to tackle the threats to health.

Today we might describe Duncan's approach as being 'strength-' or 'asset-based', recognising that for all the challenges his community was half-full, rather than half-empty, and that there were many resources available for the task if they could only be brought to the table.

APHORISM 43: ON GROWING POTATOES

You can't grow potatoes in an empty bed
(Bob Logan).

JECH, April 2002, 56: 241

FOR DISCUSSION

✦ What do you think Bob Logan meant by being unable to grow potatoes in an empty bed?

✦ What are the determinants of hospital bed occupancy?

✦ How might hospital bed occupancy be influenced by taking a whole systems approach to public health and medical care?

CASE STUDY

Irishman Bob Logan, who was an early professor of medical care at the London School of Hygiene and Tropical Medicine in the 1970s, was renowned for his aphorisms or 'Logan's Laws'. Prominent among them was his insistence that '*You can't grow potatoes in an empty bed*'.

Bob was a systems thinker who captivated his students with stories and thought-provoking aphorisms. In the days when the size of a hospital consultant's manhood was measured by the number of hospital beds that carried his name, empty beds were an anathema and patients could look forward to long lengths of stay even when their condition didn't warrant it.

Keeping your named beds fully occupied was protecting your territory. It went alongside the phenomenon of 'bed management by ward round', which for discharge purposes was often a weekly ritual, contributing to 'blocked beds' and the inefficient use of scarce resources.

This aphorism sits alongside a second of Bob's gems, namely that '*the number of [hospital] beds you have, is the number you need*'. Standing back from hospital medical care and placing it in a public health context that runs from the promotion and protection of health, self-care, primary, secondary and into specialist care and back into social care in the community, it can be seen that any health care system is perfectly designed to achieve the results it does. The neglect of public health, prevention, and self-, primary and community care produces a health care system that is unnecessarily hospital-orientated.

APHORISM 44: LIFE AND RISK

Life is a mixture of risks; what would a
risk-free life be like?

JECH, December 2005, 59: 1103

FOR DISCUSSION

+ What are the medical risks of everyday life?
+ What would a risk-free life look like?
+ What might optimal risk look like in the real world?

CASE STUDY

Daily life is not risk-free and Lowell used to say that life was a process of selecting a cause of death (Lock and Smith, 1976). It is said that one should choose one's parents wisely and the dice of life are stacked against those born into particular personal, social and environmental circumstances, even when the inherited genes are sound.

The first duty of government is to protect its citizens, but this is not without controversy and the battle for state engagement in support for health and welfare has been a long one. In liberal democracies a common goal is to enable citizens to assume some measure of control over the risks they expose themselves to.

In *Superman: The Movie*, after rescuing her from a helicopter crash, Superman reassures Lois Lane that '*flying is still the safest way to travel*', even though many people suffer from flight phobia (Ashton, 1983). Driving yourself by car is much more dangerous than flying but the key element in feeling safe is probably whether or not you are in control. When hang-gliding took off as a sport in the 1970s, the weekend news regularly reported the death of hang-gliders, but by taking control of their own sport and conducting forensic analysis of the circumstances of each fatality – weather conditions, equipment, training and errors – the sport soon became much safer.

During the heroin epidemic of the 1980s, the appearance of the human immunodeficiency virus (HIV) brought added threat and led to the implementation of syringe exchange programmes to protect injecting drug users against injections contaminated with HIV even though some argued that this was legitimising undesirable behaviour. This approach was adopted internationally and became known as '*harm reduction*' (Ashton, 2019).

APHORISM 45: THE IMPORTANCE OF HUMOUR

Humour is an essential public health skill.

JECH, July 2007, 61: 584

FOR DISCUSSION

+ Why might humour be considered as an essential prerequisite for practising public health?
+ Can you give an example of where public health has benefited from the use of humour?

CASE STUDY

Public health is concerned with serious matters of life and death and engaging the public can be difficult. It also seems to be the case that puritanical attitudes may be found among practitioners as well as libertarian.

Early in my career I found this to be the case in family planning work, perhaps more appropriately described as planned parenthood. This field seemed to attract some whose motivation was to stop certain groups from having too many babies rather than enabling women to be in charge of their reproductive destinies and life chances.

Work in public health can be seen as that of a community educator in which all the tools of the good teacher should be readily available: the ability to fill a room, to engage and entertain through storytelling and humour and by example. Coming across as a puritan can be a turn off and lead to accusations of being an adherent of the 'nanny state' rather than being a liberationist.

Humour breaks down barriers and can enable difficult topics to be addressed in a non-threatening way. According to Lowell: '*We have not considered the potential of humour in negotiation and mediation, in reducing inevitable tensions where cultural, social and political differences intersect. Humour is a lubricant that can help get us through the rough patches.*'

During one of the most important health promotion conferences of the 1980s, held in Ottawa, Canada, in 1986 (WHO et al, 1986), when some of the contributions were becoming rather 'worthy', Lowell took me out from the auditorium into a nearby shopping mall where we were able to enjoy a chunky cheeseburger as a welcome antidote.

William Shakespeare summed up the dilemma in *Twelfth Night* when Sir Toby Belch challenges Malvolio, *'Dost thou think that because thou art virtuous there shall be no more cakes and ale?'*

APHORISM 46: KILLING WITH KINDNESS

Killing with kindness: there is no defence against kindness (Sam Levin).

JECH, August 2005, 59: 644

FOR DISCUSSION

✚ From your own experience do you agree that there is no defence against kindness?

✚ If kindness is such a good way of achieving change, why do you think there is resistance to using it?

✚ Are there any limits to kindness?

CASE STUDY

How many times have you found that the way to deal with someone who is being particularly difficult in achieving a public health objective is by a concerted effort of being reasonable and keeping the agenda on an adult level?

We all bring to our work as potential change agents differing experiences from our childhood, school days and daily life of how people behave when trying to influence the world around them. If we have a scientific background we may have been led to believe that, as in the laboratory, A + B = C and that by pulling levers or adding ingredient x a predicted effect can be achieved.

However, the world in which biology interacts with society, with politics and with the environment, is very different. The rational and the irrational coexist and influence each other. Achieving change for public health is almost always about acting on a whole system rather than one of its parts.

It is said that you catch more flies with honey than with vinegar and that it is easier to change your own behaviour than somebody else's. Eric Berne, the influential author of the book *Games People Play* provides a framework for the transactional analysis of relationship dynamics (Berne, 1969). Berne describes the three fundamental roles of interpersonal interaction as those of parent, adult and child.

Each of us will have our own experiences of these roles and our own default positions when the going gets tough. As professionals we need to transcend them.

While adult–adult transactions are the most fruitful it is all too easy to play the child when somebody comes on heavy as 'parent' or to play the adult to their 'child' when they are acting out. By refusing to be drawn into the game and only offering adult behaviour, it improves the chances of getting somewhere. The implication of this is the need to be tolerant and kind when faced with provocation.

'*Killing them with kindness*' was one of Lowell's favourite aphorisms; one he attributed to his father Sam, a Beverly Hills pharmacist. It certainly can sometimes confuse people when they are looking for an argument. At the risk of mixing metaphors, it is always best to play a straight bat when faced with 'the games people play'. This is the key to building trust through consistency, a commodity that is hard to build and easy to throw away.

Are there limits to kindness? The Americans have an expression that '*your freedom ends where my nose begins*'. In the same sense it is wise to avoid witch hunts unless there are actually witches.

APHORISM 47: EVERY SILVER LINING HAS A CLOUD

Every silver lining has a cloud (Lowell S Levin).

JECH, October 2005, 59: 815

FOR DISCUSSION

✦ Can you give an example of when the light at the end of the tunnel was an oncoming train?

✦ How might you avoid the worst of the untoward consequences of public health intervention?

CASE STUDY

The law of unintended consequences – 'sod's law', or whatever you want to call it – applies to public health as to other areas of human endeavour. The Whig politicians' view of history was one of *'upwards and onwards progression towards an ever brighter future'*. Yet a reading of public health history teaches us otherwise.

In his seminal book *The Uses of Epidemiology*, post-war public health pioneer Jerry Morris identified seven uses of epidemiology: historical study; community diagnosis; calculation of individual risk; health services research; as an aid to clinical understanding; for the identification and labelling of disease; and in the search for causes. Professor Morris described a list of diseases such as rheumatic fever and appendicitis that had almost disappeared during his professional lifetime and identified others that had made a new appearance, sometimes seeming to be like peeling away the layers of an onion (Morris, 1957).

In my own time, since the 1960s, we have had to cope with and respond to a whole range of new viral and other infectious diseases including hepatitis, bovine spongiform encephalopathy (mad cow disease), HIV/AIDS, avian flu, SARS, swine flu, Ebola and Covid-19. In addition, alcohol, drug abuse, eating disorders, self-harm and other mental health issues have assumed much greater significance, together with a growing burden of disease from neurological conditions including dementia.

The Danish poet Piet Hein summed things up with his pithy 'grook' poem, '*Problems worthy of attack prove their worth by hitting back*' (Hein, 1969). Each of the classic public health problems associated with food, water and the environment may have been partially defeated only to reappear in new forms of pollution and threat as we realise the inadequacies of a mechanistic sanitary approach and the need for an ecological one rooted in sustainability.

Even significant advances, such as the discovery of insulin, may in their very efficacy create more problems by increasing the prevalence of a longstanding condition with an increased burden of disease and costs to the community. We have yet to know the cost and burden of the new disease 'Long Covid', a complication of surviving the clinical infection with the new coronavirus. This reminds us that primary prevention remains the holy grail.

Excellence in public health involves being able to make a decent shot at anticipating the unintended consequences and have follow-up strategies to mitigate those consequences.

APHORISM 48: MAKING THINGS HAPPEN

Making things happen versus watching things happening.

JECH, June 2003, 57: 394

FOR DISCUSSION

✚ Do you think of yourself mostly as somebody who feels at home in the world of ideas, as somebody who likes to get your hands dirty in the real world, or a mixture of both?

✚ In your experience, is the balance right between academic research and reflection and practical public health intervention?

✚ How might the right balance be struck to achieve public health that is characterised by 'clean minds and dirty hands'?

CASE STUDY

It is said that there are three types of person: those that make things happen, those who watch things happening and those who wonder what happened. Making things happen and acting as an agent for change is at the heart of public health practice, but so are observation and reflection.

The first UK public health observatory was set up in Liverpool in 1990 in response to growing frustration from local health authorities about their return on investment in university-based research (Ashton, 2019). The problem of conventional funding of research, intelligence and advice to the universities was due to their tendency to take the funding and disappear for several years, only to come back with the answer when the question had changed. In fast-moving public health situations, questions need to be answered in days, weeks or months rather than months and years. That first observatory was established to transform data into timely intelligence that could be the basis for practical advice.

During the 2020 Covid-19 pandemic, the UK government was criticised for allowing itself to be unduly influenced by a narrow range of theoretical academics, missing out on the experienced advice of public health practitioners who could offer clean minds and dirty hands in the face of the immense challenge posed by the novel virus and its impact on health and well-being (Ashton, 2020).

As the pandemic progressed and large-scale testing for the virus became available using lateral flow antigen tests, some public health academics were openly critical of their deployment in Liverpool to identify and self-isolate asymptomatic members of the public. Criticism centred on arguments about the sensitivity and specificity of the new tests, mistakenly equating their use with the conceptual framework underpinning screening programmes for non-communicable diseases such as breast and cervical cancer.

In practice, large-scale population testing was used to identify asymptomatic carriers of the virus and reduce its spread as a public health intervention. In the case of both Liverpool and Bahrain it achieved this dramatically in conjunction with other measures reducing infection rates from around 700 per 100,000 to under 100 in under a month (Ashton, 2020).

A balanced public health practitioner should be neither exclusively a doer, nor observer nor analyst. The artificial dichotomy between public health practice and academic life has not served us well; we need synthesis and individual and team balance. Nobody is perfect but a team can be.

It is said that John Lennon declined an invitation to take part in a debate in the Oxford Union on the grounds that he was '*only a heckler*'; but his words and music influenced a generation and arguably changed the world.

APHORISM 49: SUCCESS AND FAILURE

Success has 100 parents, failure is an orphan

JECH, December 2002, 57: 646

FOR DISCUSSION

+ Have you ever had the experience of somebody else taking the credit for your achievements? If so, was this your intention or did it leave you feeling aggrieved?
+ How might we reset our expectations such that we rejoice at others incorporating our ideas and practices and making them their own?

CASE STUDY

In the academic world we are taught that plagiarism is more or less the ultimate sin, yet in public health practice we suffer from a deficit of plagiarism and an unwillingness to do things that were 'not invented here'. Ironically the root meaning of education is to bring out from the individual, inherent knowledge and aptitude ('*educo*' – Latin, 'I lead forth, nourish, draw out').

Civil servants, on the other hand, become accustomed to hearing their own words, phrases and efforts being claimed by politicians and ministers. It is part of the job to get them there. We shouldn't be too bothered in public health practice if we don't receive the credit for our own ideas; what is important is that things happen to improve the health of the population for which we have some responsibility. The very fact of securing co-ownership will mean that frequently others claim the credit (see Aphorism 15, 'Go to the people').

The World Health Organization Healthy Cities Project, which was established in 1986, began on a small scale with 11 European cities. The WHO was keen to have a successful initiative to illustrate the implementation of the principles of the New Public Health in action and tried to keep tight control over their baby.

However, the idea of the project attracted enormous interest and acquired a life of its own to the extent that thousands of cities became involved worldwide, forming themselves into national and international networks united by a passion for the unique sense of place of each community, a universal and adaptable logo of each cityscape, and a coherent set of goals. All this was against a background bequeathed to us by those who had gone before in the form of the UK Health of Towns Association of the 1840s and President Kennedy's Model Towns Programme in the 1960s (Ashton, 1992).

Perhaps we should take a leaf from the wise parent who rejoices in offspring when they have mastered the art of riding a bicycle when they claim to have done it themselves.

APHORISM 50: THE DILEMMA OF CAPITAL CITIES

What shall we do about London?

JECH, December 2007, 61: 1019

FOR DISCUSSION

+ In what ways are capital cities unique when it comes to protecting the health of their citizens?
+ How might the strengths of capitals be optimised and their weaknesses turned into strengths?
+ How might capitals best serve the wider interests of the whole country rather than harming them through over-centralisation?

CASE STUDY

Faced with the complexity of the capital in the 1840s, Edwin Chadwick is said to have asked '*What shall we do about London?*' Since that time, health planners have often agonised about capital cities. These places are different in many ways, not least because they are on the doorstep of ministers of state who find it difficult to avoid meddling in the minutiae of everyday life, especially in health services, perhaps because of their awareness of their own potential health care needs.

For centuries people have migrated into cities, especially when they are young, and the process of rapid urbanisation that characterised the Industrial Revolution 200 years ago has become a flood with the development of mega-cities around the world. Push and pull factors have operated for more than 200 years between rural and urban areas, accelerated by technological change, war and colonial enterprise.

That process continues onwards, driven now increasingly by poverty and economic ambition, climate change and globalisation with millions of migrants travelling around the world in search of a better future for themselves and their families.

As Lowell put it, '*You have to remember they are coming here to get away from us*' – escaping the failures of the international policies of the global family of countries (JECH, September 2004, 58:765).

City life confers real benefits on many with the increased opportunity that comes from the concentration of expertise and international links, and the creaming off of talents from around the country. The downside can be social isolation and the polarisation of the rich and poor and an increasing perception that especially capital cities are leaving other places behind.

One of the originators of the WHO Healthy Cities Project, Len Duhl, who had also advised on President Kennedy's Model Towns Programme in the United States, maintained that once cities exceeded populations of more than 250,000–500,000 their governance became much more problematic (Ashton, 1992). Duhl held that above this size it was necessary to devolve functions to the organic entities that make up the whole.

For most cities this will involve the historic villages and suburban centres that have coalesced to form the metropolitan area following principles of subsidiarity and additionality, in that functions should be carried out as near to people as makes sense not only financially but also from the point of view of citizen coherence. Functions should be carried out for the whole city only if they cannot be carried out efficiently and coherently at the more proximal level.

In the aftermath of the 2020 Covid-19 pandemic, radical changes are in prospect with rebalancing of the work–life balance, potential flight from the cities to smaller, more manageable and greener environments, and an increasing imperative to address the extreme social inequalities that have been allowed to develop in recent decades.

REFERENCES

Adams, D (1979) *The Hitchhiker's Guide to the Galaxy*. London: Pan Books.

Antonovsky, A (1987) *Unravelling the Mystery of Health: How People Manage Stress and Stay Well*. San Francisco, CA: Jossey-Bass.

Ashton, J (1983) Risk Assessment. *British Medical Journal*, 286: 1843.

Ashton, J (1992) *Healthy Cities*. Milton Keynes: Open University Press.

Ashton, J (2019) *Practising Public Health: An Eyewitness Account*. Oxford: Oxford University Press.

Ashton, J (2020) *Blinded by Corona: How the Pandemic Ruined Britain's Health and Wealth*. London: Gibson Square Press.

Ashton, J and Seymour, H (1989) *The New Public Health*. Milton Keynes: Open University Press.

Barry, J M (2004) *The Great Influenza: The Epic Story of the Deadliest Plague in History*. New York, NY: Viking Press.

Baum, L F (1900) *The Wonderful Wizard of Oz*. Chicago, IL: George M Hill Company.

Berne, E (1969) *Games People Play: The Psychology of Human Relationships*. New York, NY: Grove Press.

Carson, R (1962) *Silent Spring*. Boston, MA: Houghton Mifflin.

Chadwick, E (1964 [1842]) *Report on the Sanitary Condition of the Labouring Population of Great Britain*, ed M W Finn. Edinburgh: Edinburgh University Press.

Donaldson, L (2002) *An Organisation with a Memory: Report of an Expert Group on Learning from Adverse Events in the NHS Chaired by the Chief Medical Officer*. London: The Stationery Office.

Durkheim, E (1975) *Suicide: A Study in Sociology*. London: Routledge and Kegan Paul.

Durrell, L (1960) Landscape and Character. *The New York Times*, 12 June.

Frazer, W M (1947) *Duncan of Liverpool: An Account of the Work of Dr W. H. Duncan, Medical Officer of Health of Liverpool, 1847–63*. London: Hamish Hamilton.

Friedson, E (1970) *Profession of Medicine: A Study of the Sociology of Applied Knowledge*. Chicago, IL: University of Chicago Press.

Gladwell, M (2000) *The Tipping Point: How Little Things Can Make a Big Difference*. Boston, MA: Little, Brown.

Hein, P (1969) *Grooks*. London: Hodder and Stoughton.

Iacobucci, G (2020) Covid-19: Doctors are Given New Guidelines on When to Admit Patients to Critical Care. *British Medical Journal*, 368: m1189.

Illich, I (1974) *Medical Nemesis: The Expropriation of Health*. London: Calder and Boyars.

Kickbusch, I, Allen, L and Franz, C (2016) The Commercial Determinants of Health. *The Lancet*, 4(12): E895–6.

Kretzmann, J P and McKnight, J L (1993) *Building Communities from the Inside Out: A Path toward Finding and Mobilising a Community's Assets*. Evanston, IL: Asset Based Community Development Institute.

Levin, L S and Adler, E L (1981) *The Hidden Health Care System: Mediating Structures and Medicine*. Cambridge, MA: Ballinger Publishing Company.

Lock, S and Smith, T (1976) *The Medical Risks of Life*. London: Penguin Books.

Marmot, M, Goldblatt, P and Allen, J (2010) *Fair Society, Healthy Lives: The Marmot Review*. London: Institute of Health Equity.

McBane, J (2008) *The Rebirth of Liverpool: The Eldonian Way*. Liverpool: Liverpool University Press.

McKeown, T (1976) *The Role of Medicine: Dream, Mirage or Nemesis?* London: Nuffield Provincial Hospitals Trust.

McKnight, J (1995) *The Careless Society: Community and its Counterfeits*. New York, NY: Basic Books.

McKnight, J and Block, P (2010) *The Abundant Community: Awakening the Power of Families and Neighbourhoods*. San Francisco: American Planning Association and Berrett-Koehler Publishers.

Mental Health Foundation (2016) *Better Mental Health for All: A Public Health Approach to Mental Health Improvement*. London: Faculty of Public Health and Mental Health Foundation.

Mill, J S (1859) *On Liberty*. London: John W. Parker and Son.

Morris, J N (1957) *The Uses of Epidemiology*. Edinburgh and London: Churchill Livingstone.

Seedhouse, D (2001) *Health: The Foundations of Achievement*. New York, NY: Wiley.

Sigerist, H E (1941) *Medicine and Human Welfare*. New Haven, CT: Yale University Press.

Shaw, G B (1906) *The Doctor's Dilemma*. London: Royal Court Theatre.

Snow, C P (1959) *The Two Cultures*. Cambridge: Cambridge University Press.

Susser, M (1973) *Causal Thinking in the Health Sciences*. Oxford: Oxford University Press.

United Nations (2015) *Transforming Our World: The 2030 Agenda for Sustainable Development*. New York, NY: United Nations.

Watson, J D (1968) *The Double Helix*. New York: Simon and Schuster.

Wilczek, F (2015) Einstein's Parable of Quantum Insanity. *Quanta Magazine*, 23 September.

Winslow, C E A (1920) The Untilled Fields of Public Health. *Science*, 51(1306): 23–33.

Wohl, A S (1984) *Endangered Lives: Public Health in Victorian Britain*. London: Methuen.

World Commission on Environment and Development (WCED) (1987) *Our Common Future*. Oxford: Oxford University Press.

World Health Organization (WHO) (1946) *Constitution*. Geneva: WHO.

World Health Organization (WHO) (1981) *Global Strategy for Health for All by the Year 2000*. Geneva: WHO.

World Health Organization (WHO) (2002) *World Report on Violence and Health*. Geneva: WHO.

World Health Organization (WHO), Health and Welfare Canada and Canadian Public Health Association (1986) *Ottawa Charter for Health Promotion*. Copenhagen: WHO.

INDEX